Clinical Context for Evidence-Based Nursing Practice

The *Evidence-Based Nursing Series*

The *Evidence-Based Nursing Series* is co-published with Sigma Theta Tau International (STTI). The series focuses on implementing evidence-based practice in nursing and mirrors the remit of *Worldviews on Evidence-Based Nursing*, encompassing clinical practice, administration, research and public policy.

Other titles in the *Evidence-Based Nursing Series*:

Models and Frameworks for Implementing Evidence-Based Practice: Linking Evidence to Action
Edited by Jo Rycroft-Malone and Tracey Bucknall
ISBN: 978-1-4051-7594-4

Evaluating the Impact of Implementing Evidence-Based Practice
Edited by Debra Bick and Ian D. Graham
ISBN: 978-1-4051-8384-0

Clinical Context for Evidence-Based Nursing Practice

Edited by

Bridie Kent
Professor of Nursing Eastern Health-Deakin University,
Melbourne, Victoria, Australia

and

Brendan McCormack
Professor of Nursing Research
Institute of Nursing Research/School of Nursing,
University of Ulster, Northern Ireland

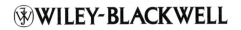

WILEY-BLACKWELL

A John Wiley & Sons, Ltd., Publication

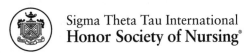

Sigma Theta Tau International
Honor Society of Nursing®

This edition first published 2010
© 2010 Sigma Theta Tau International

Blackwell Publishing was acquired by John Wiley & Sons in February 2007.
Blackwell's publishing programme has been merged with Wiley's global Scientific,
Technical, and Medical business to form Wiley-Blackwell.

Registered office
John Wiley & Sons Ltd, The Atrium, Southern Gate, Chichester, West Sussex,
PO19 8SQ, United Kingdom

Editorial offices
9600 Garsington Road, Oxford, OX4 2DQ, United Kingdom
2121 State Avenue, Ames, Iowa 50014-8300, USA

For details of our global editorial offices, for customer services and for information
about how to apply for permission to reuse the copyright material in this book
please see our website at www.wiley.com/wiley-blackwell.

The right of the author to be identified as the author of this work has been asserted
in accordance with the UK Copyright, Designs and Patents Act 1988.

Library of Congress Cataloging-in-Publication Data
Clinical context for evidence-based nursing practice / edited by
Bridie Kent and Brendan McCormack.
   p. ; cm. — (Evidence-based nursing series)
Includes bibliographical references and index.
ISBN 978-1-4051-8433-5 (pbk. : alk. paper)
1. Evidence-based nursing. 2. Context effects (Psychology) I. Kent,
Bridie. II. McCormack, Brendan. III. Series: Evidence-based nursing series.
[DNLM: 1. Evidence-Based Nursing—methods. 2. Clinical Competence.
WY 100.7 C641 2010]
RT84.5.C567 2010
610.73—dc22
2010007737

A catalogue record for this book is available from the British Library.

Set in 11/13 pt Sabon by MPS Limited, A Macmillan Company
Printed and bound in Malaysia by Vivar Printing Sdn Bhd

1   2010

Contents

Foreword

Over more years than seems possible, I spent considerable time and energy in various medical centers attempting to facilitate and evaluate evidence-based practice (EBP) and organizational innovation efforts. This experience and related evaluative data increasingly highlighted for me the importance of the context within which enthusiastic nurses tried to implement change. For such change to be successful, which includes change that is sustained over time, and to move beyond individual enthusiasm or organizational "adoption in principle," the critical nature of contextual factors had to be recognized and actively addressed.

This book in the EBP Series on the role of context provides validation for the above observation; and it is significant for anyone interested in truly "making EBP happen" in practice, in any country. Its content provides an overview of the meaning, complexity, and criticality of context. It demonstrates the universality of contextual impact on EBP across specialty areas and multiple types of practice settings. It provides real life examples, describes suggested implementation approaches, and highlights the existence of research on this issue within nursing—as well as the need for more research within nursing on the relationship of context, implementation approaches, and actualization of EBP. It provides paradigms and theories for consideration, as well as links to additional resources to enhance readers' knowledge and skills on the subject. In the end, it draws attention to the fact that reflective practitioners interested in enhancing the quality of care they and their colleagues deliver need to knowledgably reflect upon, assess and influence the context in which they hope to make adoption of EBP a reality.

Cheryl B. Stetler, PhD, RN, FAAN

Cover Image

The 'tantrix puzzle' image of the book cover represents the complexity of the concept of 'practice context' and the depth of levels at which contextual characteristics operate. Increasingly, researchers in the field of knowledge translation recognise that context is a complex issue and that it has significant influence over the way in which knowledge is used in practice. Like the tantrix puzzle, unravelling the elements of context requires an understanding of how the different components of a practice setting connect with each other. Each connection influences the shape and position of the next and it is only through working out the logic of the connections can the puzzle be solved—or context be understood.

Notes on contributors

Tracey Bucknall

Tracey Bucknall PhD, Grad Dip Adv Nurs, BN, ICU Cert, RN is currently Professor, School of Nursing, Deakin University and Head, Cabrini-Deakin Centre for Nursing Research, Cabrini Health, Australia, and is an Associate Editor of *Worldviews on Evidence-Based Nursing*.

During her career, Tracey has held a variety of clinical, educational, and research appointments in both private and public hospitals, and in the tertiary sector. Tracey's primary research interests are clinical decision making and implementation of research into practice. Her research focuses on understanding how individuals make decisions routinely and in uncertainty, the environmental and social influences encountered in changing contexts, and interventions to improve the uptake of research in practice. More recently she has incorporated patient involvement in decision making as a means of influencing clinician uptake of research evidence.

Jane Cahill

Jane Cahill (MA Hons; PhD) is Research Fellow at the School of Healthcare, University of Leeds. She has extensive experience of psychological therapy effectiveness research having worked for the Psychological Therapies Research Centre at the University of Leeds for nine years before being appointed to the School of Healthcare. Her current programme of research supports the mental health research stream within the school and has a particular focus on the therapeutic alliance, practice-based evidence approaches, workforce mental health issues, and complementary and alternative approaches to mental health.

Dawn Freshwater

Dawn Freshwater PhD, BA, UKCP Reg, RGN, FRCN is Professor of Mental Health and Head of the School of Healthcare, University of Leeds. Her research interests span across mental health, prison healthcare, and psychosocial interventions. She is keen to examine and develop innovative ways of understanding and implementing research within the healthcare system and has used a variety of post-modern approaches to underpin her research grant activity. She is the author of 15 books, has contributed widely to academic discourse around research methods, and is currently the editor of the *Journal of Psychiatric Mental Health Nursing*. She is a Fellow of the Royal College of Nursing and a registered psychotherapist.

Gill Harvey

Gill Harvey PhD, BNurs, is a Reader in Health Management at Manchester Business School (MBS). She has a professional background in nursing and, prior to taking up post at MBS, Gill worked for 9 years as the Director of the Royal College of Nursing's Quality Improvement Programme. Whilst working at the RCN, Gill was also responsible for establishing and leading the National Collaborating Centre for Nursing and Supportive Care, funded by the National Institute for Health and Clinical Excellence (NICE), to develop clinical guidelines for the NHS. Gill's research interests are focused on two main areas: organizational failure and turnaround and evaluative research around issues of implementation and facilitating quality improvement in practice.

Alison Hutchinson

Alison Hutchinson PhD, MBioeth, BAppSc (Adv Nsg), Midwifery Certificate, Nursing Certificate is currently Associate Professor at Deakin University and Cabrini Health, Australia. Following completion of a hospital-based nursing education, Alison undertook a Bachelor of Applied Science (Advanced Nursing) at La Trobe University, Melbourne, Australia. In 1991 she completed midwifery certificate training at the Mercy Hospital for Women in Melbourne. In 1996 she fulfilled the requirements for the award of Master of Bioethics at Monash University, Melbourne, and in 2004, supported by Australian Research Council, Strategic Partnership in Research Training Award; she completed a Doctorate in Philosophy at The University of Melbourne. Her PhD research examined research utilization by nurses in the context of a multidisciplinary setting. In July 2007 she was awarded CIHR and AHFMR Postdoctoral Fellowships and commenced her fellowship under the supervision of Dr Carole Estabrooks at the University of Alberta. Her postdoctoral work has focused on the influence of context and interdisciplinary interaction on the uptake of research evidence by health professionals.

Nadine Janes

Nadine Janes PhD, MSc, ACNP(cert), GNC(C), RN has been a gerontological nurse for more than 20 years. She has worked as an unregulated care provider, a registered nurse, and an advanced practice nurse in both institutional and community settings. Currently, Nadine holds positions across academia and practice. She is the Manager of Professional Practice at West Park Healthcare Centre as well as an Adjunct Professor at Ryerson University, both in Toronto, Canada. Through her research Nadine is exploring the process by which nursing staff utilize knowledge about best practice when caring for older persons in aged care settings. As a clinical leader in a rehabilitation and complex continuing care setting, she has the opportunity to apply, test, and refine her research findings at the point-of-care on a day-to-day basis. Finally, through her teaching, Nadine educates tomorrow's nursing leaders about the complexities involved in supporting nurses to do what they know is best in moments of practice.

Bridie Kent

Bridie Kent PhD, BSc(Hons), PGCert Teaching in HE, RNT, RN, FCNA(NZ) is the Professor at Deakin University and Chair of Nursing at Eastern Health. She leads the Eastern Health Nursing and Midwifery Research Unit, Melbourne, Australia. Over the last two decades, Bridie has held clinical and academic appointments that have provided her with opportunities to link research, education, and practice in three different healthcare settings—UK, New Zealand, and Australia. She has over 15 years of experience in the field of critical care, been leading research-based teaching in this area of practice, and has contributed to a number of key texts, all of which help to inform and guide decision making in clinical practice. She is an experienced nurse researcher, with extensive experience in quality improvement, practice change, health services education, and research in the UK, New Zealand, and Australia, using associations with other leading centers to achieve sustainable results. For the last 8 years, she has played a leading role in evidence-based practice uptake and implementation in New Zealand, and through the Joanna Briggs Collaboration, helped to advance the science of evidence-based practice internationally. She is the Director of the Deakin Centre for Quality and Risk Management: A collaborating centre of the Joanna Briggs Institute. She is also Associate Editor of *Implementation Science* and Section Editor of *Worldviews on Evidence-Based Nursing*.

Debbie Kralik

Debbie Kralik RN, PhD is General Manager of Strategy and Research at the Royal District Nursing Service in South Australia. She is Adjunct Associate Professor at the University of South Australia and Adelaide University. Her research interests for the past decade have been the experience of chronic illness and community care. Debbie is Senior Editor of two journals: the *Journal of Advanced Nursing* and the *Journal of Nursing and Healthcare of Chronic Illness*.

Brendan McCormack

Brendan McCormack D.Phil (Oxon.), BSc (Hons.), PGCEA, RNT, RMN, RGN is currently the Professor of Nursing Research, Institute of Nursing Research/School of Nursing, University of Ulster, Northern Ireland; Adjunct Professor of Nursing, University of Technology, Sydney; Adjunct Professor of Nursing, Faculty of Medicine, Nursing and Health Care, Monash University, Melbourne.

He leads a number of practice development and research projects in Ireland, the UK, Europe, and Australia, which focus on the development of person-centered practice. In addition he is the Head of the Person-centred Practice Research Centre in the Institute of Nursing Research, coordinating research and development activity in this area. His writing and research work focuses on gerontological nursing, person-centered nursing, and practice development, and he serves on a number of editorial boards, policy committees, and development groups in these areas. He is the editor of the *International Journal of Older People Nursing*. He has coauthored *Practice Development in Nursing* which has now been translated into two languages and *Practice Development in Nursing: International Perspectives*. Brendan is Chair of the Older Person's Charity, AgeNI and President of the All-Ireland Gerontological Nurses Association (AIGNA).

John Rosenberg

John Rosenberg PhD, RN holds a Teaching and Research position in the University of Queensland School of Nursing and Midwifery and was the Chair of Palliative Care Nurses Australia Inc. from 2008 to 2010. He is a registered nurse with a clinical background in community-based palliative care. He has also worked as an educator and researcher in the care of people at the end of life. John was conferred a PhD by Queensland University of Technology in 2007, which examined the integration of health promotion principles and practice in palliative care organizations. John's ongoing scholarly interests lie in sociological perspectives of death and dying and in the engagement of palliative care organizations with the wider community in the support of people at the end of life. John is also interested in the promotion of advanced skills in palliative care nursing and is a coauthor of the Competency Standards for Specialist Palliative Care Nursing Practice.

Marlene Sinclair

Marlene Sinclair's PhD MEd DASE BSc RNT RM RN, Specialist certificate in Neuromedicine/Neurosurgery career highlights have been in midwifery education and research. Marlene holds a personal chair for Midwifery Research at the Institute of Nursing Research, University of Ulster and is President and founder of the Doctoral Midwifery Research Society. Her specialist area of research is the appropriate use of technology in childbirth and her work extends from Ireland, to the UK and further afield to Taiwan and Jordan. She is editor and founder of the Royal College of Midwives (RCM) research journal, Evidence Based Midwifery.

Victoria M. Steelman

Victoria Steelman PhD, RN, CNOR, FAAN is an Assistant Professor at the College of Nursing, The University of Iowa, in Iowa City, IA, USA. She focused on implementing evidence-based practice changes in perioperative settings for 20 years. She has published extensively and presented about issues related to safe patient care in the operating room and authored many of the Association of periOperative Registered Nurses Recommended Practices. She is well recognized for these activities and received two Outstanding Achievement awards from the AORN for this work. In 2007, she was inducted into the American Academy of Nursing in recognition of the national and global impact of her work. In 2008, she received AORN's highest honor, the Award for Excellence in recognition of her contributions to perioperative nursing.

Valerie Wilson

Valerie Wilson PhD, MN, Bed St., RSCN, RN is the Director of Nursing Research & Practice Development at the Children's Hospital at Westmead and Professor of Nursing Research & Practice Development at the University of Technology, Sydney. She has extensive experience in practice development, facilitation, and evaluation. She completed her PhD in 2005, in which she evaluated the effectiveness of practice development strategies in a Special Care Nursery. The results of her research have been published in several nursing and practice development journals and books.

She is member of a Knowledge Utilization/Translation group as well as the International Practice Development collaborative. Her focus is on working with clinicians to develop person-centered approaches to care, that are both evidence based and take into account the needs of patients and families. The evaluation of this work, together with a number of local, state, and international projects form the basis of her research work.

Chapter 1

Introduction

Bridie Kent and Brendan McCormack

Evidence-informed practice has, in the western world, been the driver for many changes in nursing education, policy, and research. As Ciliska (2006) indicated it is now accepted as the norm "Every nurse should have at least an understanding of the purpose and process of evidence-based practice, be able to ask relevant clinical questions, and know who in their environment can assist them in answering questions." (p. 38). Concerns over adverse events, quality of care, and the quest for clinical effectiveness have led to guides, books, and decision-aids being developed to assist nurses, and other health professionals, with the utilization of evidence in their practice.

Implementation of evidence is a science in its own right, and is associated with specific challenges. One of these relates to the detailed knowledge and skills that health professionals have been encouraged to learn and adopt. The plethora of published works (research and textbooks) is testament to the attention that evidence-informed healthcare has attracted over recent years. This series adds further to the toolkit of resources available for use by health professionals.

So, there is no shortage of resources but what is lacking is a sound understanding of the issues that positively or negatively influence the uptake of evidence into practice. Increasingly, the importance of "context" as a key influence on the translation and use of evidence in practice is recognized. However, context is not a simple concept; the multifaceted nature of the factors related to context raises a variety of challenges to the systematic implementation of evidence into practice. This complexity has resulted in context being referred to by many knowledge translation researchers as "the black-box of practice"

(Rycroft-Malone, 2007). Despite many years of research into evidence-based practice, knowledge utilization, and knowledge translation, we continue to know very little about what makes a context receptive to evidence, what contextual factors have the most impact on clinical effectiveness and clinical decision making, what interventions work best to change practice context, and possibly the most challenging of all—how best to evaluate changes in practice context. Thus there is a clear need for ongoing research in this field to clarify the concept and to develop methods for assessing and appraising the potential impact of individual contextual factors on evidence implementation and the resulting impact of context on implementation interventions.

McCormack et al. (2002) highlighted the variability of contexts in which healthcare takes place and the breadth of factors that subsequently influence practice settings. The context of healthcare can be seen, on one level, as infinite as it takes place in a variety of settings, communities, and cultures that are all influenced by a variety of factors, for example, sociocultural, political, economic, and historical factors. However, in their concept analysis of context, McCormack et al. (2002) used the term to refer to the environment or setting in which people receive healthcare services, or in the context of getting research evidence into practice, "the environment or setting in which the proposed change is to be implemented" (Kitson et al., 1998). They suggested that, in its most simple form, context refers to the physical environment in which practice takes place. Whilst this may seem like an oversimplistic idea, having some boundaried understanding of context is important. In particular, international evidence suggests that nurses have a strong allegiance with the setting in which they work (e.g., a ward, department, clinic, community) (Aiken et al., 2001) and less so with an organization at large and thus the systems, structures, processes, and patterns in an organization are experienced differently in particular practice settings. The boundary of the practice setting shapes how a clinician experiences the organization and, ultimately, how such things as evidence are translated into practice. With this notion of a boundaried practice environment in mind, McCormack et al. (2002) identified three characteristics of context—culture, leadership, and evaluation.

The literature on culture in health and social care is complex, broad, and diverse. Manley (2004) has argued that some of the problems associated with understanding culture arise from a lack of distinction in the literature (and among decision makers) between "organizational culture" and "workplace culture." Davies et al. (2000) argue that whilst there are many conceptions of culture, broadly speaking perspectives are divided between those that view culture as something an organization "is" and those that view it as something that an organization "has." The former being characteristics that are "fixed," immutable, and serve as descriptors of an organization. When an organization is considered to "have" culture then these are "aspects or variables of the organisation that can be isolated, described and manipulated" (p. 112). Davies et al. (2000) also purport that it is only through the view that organizations "have culture" that it is possible to consider ways in which culture can be changed. Manley (2004), however, argues that organizations are cultures, incorporating such things as language, myths, rules, and stories. However, Manley suggests that this (organizational culture) is not the culture that patients and staff experience everyday, instead, what they do experience is the culture of different settings (contexts) or workplaces. Wilson et al., (2005), Coeling and Simms (1993), and Adams and Bond (1997) have all argued that there is a need to understand the culture of the individual workplace prior to implementing innovations or developments, as culture has been found to vary between units within the same organization. An effective workplace culture is one in which there is (Manley, 2004, p. 2):

- a person-centered approach with patients, users, and staff;
- daily decision making that is transparent and evidence-based, where evidence is the blending of different sources of knowledge (patient preferences, empirical research, critical reflection of experience and professional expertise, and local knowledge [e.g., audit findings]);
- a learning culture in which through formal critique there is a focus on individual, team, and service effectiveness;
- development of leadership potential to achieve a culture of empowerment, continuing modernization and innovation.

The impact of leaders, and leadership roles and styles in particular, has been shown to be a significant factor in shaping culture and the context of practice. There is a large and diverse literature espousing the virtues and otherwise of particular leadership roles and styles. In modern healthcare, much emphasis is placed on "transformational leadership." Transformational leaders create a culture that recognizes everybody as a leader of something. They inspire staff toward a shared vision of some future state, as well as a number of other processes such as challenging and stimulating, enabling, developing trust, and communicating. Transformational leaders require emotional intelligence, rationality, motivational skills, empathy, and inspirational qualities and the intellectual qualities of strategic sensing, analytical skills, and self-confidence in public presentation (Kouzes & Posner, 1993). Schein (1985) suggests that transformational leaders can transpose their individual beliefs and values into collective beliefs and values and that these eventually become assumptions because they are seen to work reliably and then are taken for granted. Thus, it is implied that the transformational leader can alter the dominant practice culture and create a context that is more conducive to the integration of evidence and practice. Transformational leaders can facilitate the integration of the "science" component of healthcare practice (the application of science and technology) and the "art" component (the translation of different forms of practice knowledge) to enable the development of expertise in practice and a shared understanding of knowledge for practice. However, whilst such integration enables greater effectiveness in practice, it raises challenges in terms of evaluating practice effectiveness, the effectiveness of interventions, and patient outcomes.

Evaluating outcomes from practice is essential to healthcare effectiveness and in everyday practice is manifested through medical audit, clinical audit, standard setting, quality improvement programmes, care pathway monitoring, and accreditation. However it is widely recognized that measuring effectiveness is complex and the answering of one effectiveness question raises many others and, indeed, most effectiveness evaluation can only ever "partially answer" questions. Whilst the "hard" data of cost-effectiveness and resource management provide a particular perspective on the effectiveness of practice, if we believe that an effective workplace culture is multifaceted and multilayered, as described earlier, then the evaluation of these perspectives and layers is also important. Thus, the "hard" outcome data that can inform the effectiveness of particular interventions and the "soft" data of user experiences, staff feedback, peer review, and reflections on practice are equally valid.

A good example of the influence of contextual factors on evidence uptake is found when the practice of preoperative fasting is explored. Despite high quality evidence-based guidelines, such as those issued by the UK's Royal College of Nursing (2005), many patients continue to suffer unduly from dehydration, delayed healing, and other complications. Lorch (2007) explored the implementation of these guidelines in the orthopedic setting and identified barriers to their uptake, which included:

- resistance from theater staff and a few consultant surgeons
- difficulty educating night staff
- rapid turnover of domestic staff
- fear from junior doctors and nursing staff of upsetting the surgeons' routines
- lack of awareness by nursing staff of free space on morning elective lists.

Here we have evidence of attitudinal, environmental, economic, and communication factors that combine in various ways resulting in poor application of evidence within clinical practice settings and the adverse effects experienced by patients.

So what can be done?

Education or the presence of clinical guidelines, as a sole activity, is insufficient to change health professionals' behavior (Grimshaw et al., 2004). A greater understanding is needed, supplemented by practice examples, and that is what we hope to achieve with this book. Experts in evidence-based practice and knowledge translation have summarized the key contextual factors that impact positively and negatively on practice change in their various healthcare settings. There will be some overlap but we make no apologies for this. It is useful to understand that there are some common contextual influences, while others tend to be setting or field specific.

There are some guides to assist evidence implementation or knowledge translation, the latter of which is the term currently favored by many implementation scientists and is widely used as a key word in articles published in many leading journals (Kent et al., 2009). Understanding how knowledge is translated into practice is important; it focuses on methods or processes that can be used to increase clinicians' practice-related knowledge and how they can use that knowledge to improve patient outcomes or health services to close or lessen the evidence-practice gap (Westbrook & Gagnon, 2009).

This brief overview of context and the way it is understood in the context of this book highlights the need for different perspectives of practice context to be brought together into one volume and to analyze how these perspectives help shape our thinking. It is for this reason that we have asked different experts in the field of evidence-based practice to comment on and discuss the contextual factors that commonly affect the uptake or utilization of evidence by practitioners. Implementation scientists have to consider differences in settings, organizational factors, the variability in cultures that exist within practice settings and all the other external and internal influences such as micro-, meso- and macroeconomics, environment, history, and politics. Add to these individual psychosocial factors such as attitudes, beliefs, and knowledge and the complexity of context as a mediating factor for successful evidence implementation becomes acutely apparent.

In Chapter 2, context is explored further by drawing on relevant models and theories that will help to develop an overview of the work that has been taking place in terms of conceptualizing contextual factors that affect evidence-based practice. By no means is this overview comprehensive and all-encompassing; that was not the aim of this chapter. What it does is highlight the common contextual factors that have been identified over the past decade or so and provide possible tools for use when considering implementing evidence into practice.

In Chapter 3, the contextual factors associated with primary care settings are explored, using examples of studies conducted within this setting. Debbie Kralik and John Rosenberg have many years of primary care experience between them, and they have worked in a variety of settings including district nursing and community palliative care.

Chapter 4 moves the exploration to the other extreme of care provision; the acute care sector. Alison Hutchinson and Tracey Bucknall draw on implementation projects that they and others have conducted to capture the key contextual factors that commonly impact on knowledge translation in the acute care setting. Alison and Tracey both hold joint clinical and academic appointments and actively engage in the promotion and uptake of evidence-based practice on a daily basis.

Pediatrics forms the focus of Chapter 5. Val Wilson, an experienced pediatric registered nurse, also draws on research conducted by herself and others to provide examples of how contextual factors can positively and negatively influence knowledge translation and practice change. She uses work conducted in the special care nursery environment to illustrate key factors related to embedding evidence into practice, and also reveals how problems arising in practice can be addressed by research and practice change to reflect new evidence.

Chapter 6 takes the reader to the specialised perioperative setting. Victoria Steelman has extensive expertise infusing evidence-based practice into healthcare settings and has a particular interest in studying safety and quality. She has made significant contributions to perioperative nursing, in the USA and further afield, and once again, she draws on her research to provide an overview of the factors that should be considered when undertaking knowledge translation activities in the perioperative setting.

We move to another specialist field of healthcare, Midwifery, in Chapter 7. Marlene Sinclair, who is Ireland's first Professor of Midwifery Research, draws on her research experiences, particularly in birth technology, that span both qualitative and quantitative methods. She captures the contextual factors that are associated with Midwifery practice and includes examples that will not only enhance our understanding of issues in this area of practice but also our knowledge and understanding of technology in the birthing process and birth outcomes.

Mental health is the focus of Chapter 8. Dawn Freshwater and Jane Cahill explore the context of evidence as developed and applied in mental healthcare settings. In particular, they draw on two examples of how evidence can be used to both define and influence practice environments and subsequently impact on care; the process of benchmarking and the practice of reviewing research and research evidence.

In Chapter 9 the focus shifts to the care of older persons. In a world where people are generally living longer and healthier lives, it is important to explore how to provide the best in healthcare for older persons. Nadine Janes has a wealth of experience to draw on; she has worked as an unregulated care provider, a registered nurse, and as an advanced practice nurse in both institutional and community settings. Therefore she is extremely well placed to consider the aged care setting, in particular the factors that affect knowledge translation in long-term care facilities.

We move from the specific to the wider world in Chapter 10. Gill Harvey explores issues relating to the wider policy context of implementation, looking in particular at the relationships between policy and practice in relation to delivering evidence-based healthcare.

She discusses the factors that influence decision making at a policy level and draws on specific examples to illustrate how the policy process can mediate the translation of evidence into practice, pushing some issues higher up the agenda and others lower down.

We know that we have not included all settings or fields of practice; that would be virtually impossible in a book of this size. We also recognize that many of the examples are from the western world and few from the rapidly developing eastern societies. By exploring context in various clinical settings, we hope that the factors will be seen in such a way that they can be transferred to other settings that we have not covered and similarly be considered when undertaking knowledge translation in any part of the world. In the final chapter we will synthesise the key issues emerging from previous chapters and propose some options for moving forward with advancing our knowledge of context and identifying future research priorities in this field.

We will begin however with the next chapter, which provides an overview of context, and draws on frameworks or models that can be used by health professionals to identify and assess the impact that each has on achieving successful practice change.

References

Adams, A. & Bond, S. (1997). Clinical specialty and organizational features of acute hospital wards. *Journal of Advanced Nursing*, 26, 1158–1167.

Aiken, H., Clarke, S.P., Sloane, D.M. et al. (2001). Nurses reports on hospital are in five countries. *Health Affairs—Web Exclusive*, 20, 45–53.

Ciliska, D. (2006). Evidence-based nursing: How far have we come? What's next? *Evidence-Based Nursing*, 9, 38–40.

Coeling, H. & Simms, L. (1993). Facilitating innovation at the unit level through cultural assessment, Part 2: Adapting managerial ideas to the unit work group. *Journal of Nursing Administration*, 23, 13–20.

Davies, H.T.O., Nutley, S.M. & Mannion, R. (2000). Organisational culture and quality of health care. *Quality in Health Care*, 9, 111–119.

Grimshaw, J., Thomas, R., Maclennan, G. et al. (2004). Effectiveness and efficiency of guidelines dissemination and implementation strategies. *Health Technology Assessment*, 8(6), 1–72.

Kent, B., Hutchinson, A.M. & Fineout-Overholt, E. (2009). Getting evidence into practice—understanding knowledge translation to achieve practice change. *Worldviews on Evidence-Based Nursing*, 6, 183–185.

Kitson, A., Harvey, G. & McCormack, B. (1998). Approaches to implementing research in practice. *Quality in Health Care*, 7, 149–159.

Kouzes, J. & Posner, B. (1993). Transformational leadership. The credibility factor. *The Healthcare Forum Journal*, 36, 16–24.

Lorch, A. (2007). Implementation of fasting guidelines through nursing leadership. *Nursing Times*, 103, 30–31.

Manley, K. (2004). Transformational culture: A culture of effectiveness. In: Mccormack, B., Manley, K. & Garbett, R. (eds) *Practice Development in Nursing*. Oxford: Blackwell.

McCormack, B., Kitson, A., Harvey, G., Rycroft-Malone, J., Titchen, A. & Seers, K. (2002). Getting evidence into practice: The meaning of "context." *Journal of Advanced Nursing*, 38, 94–104.

Royal College of Nursing (2005). Perioperative fasting in adults and children: An RCN guideline for the multidisciplinary team. London: Royal College of Nursing.

Rycroft-Malone, J. (2007). Theory and knowledge translation: Setting some co-ordinates? *Nursing Research*, 56, 578–585.

Schein, E.H. (1985). *Organizational Culture and Leadership*. San Francisco: Jossey-Bass.

Westbrook, J. & Gagnon, M. (2009). Knowledge translation initiative for DBTACs. Austin, TX: National Center for the Dissemination of Disability Research (NCDDR)/SEDL.

Wilson, V., McCormack, B. & Ives, G. (2005). Understanding the workplace culture of a special care nursery. *Journal of Advanced Nursing*, 50, 27–38.

Chapter 2

Context: overview and application

Bridie Kent and Brendan McCormack

Introduction

This chapter will look at the different definitions and understandings of "context" and explore what this includes from different perspectives. The models and frameworks that specifically mention context will be explored further, with clarification of the similarities or differences between them and how they have been used. Also included is a discussion of the ways of approaching the critical appraisal of contextual issues in relation to evidence-based practice. Readers will be "sign-posted" to the other books of this series that explore models and approaches to support evidence implementation, and assessing the outcomes of implementation, respectively.

Defining context

Evidence-based practice has, since the late 1990s, become a driving force for problem-solving to improve clinical practice and cost-effectiveness of care (Fineout-Overholt et al., 2004). Many healthcare organizations have invested heavily in strategies to increase the likelihood that all clinical practice is evidence based wherever possible, thus moving practice away from a reliance upon rituals. The drive for improvements in quality and effectiveness in healthcare and the need to enhance patient safety, which have triggered the rapid growth in evidence-based practice resources, have required a change in culture, away from paternalistic care provision, to one of person-centered care in which the practitioner is a critical thinking, reflective, knowledge-based doer. By utilizing approaches that raise awareness of taken-for-granted assumptions and then critically reflecting on these, a greater understanding of both practice and the evidence available for use in practice emerges. Awareness of the importance of the context in which evidence-based practice takes place also emerges. It is through critical reflection around the use of research findings that health professionals can understand more fully the internal and external contexts of the practice setting in which adoption of evidence is being considered. With this knowledge, the likelihood of successful delivery of evidence-based person-centered care may be maximized.

Although many readers will be aware of the history of EBP, it does no harm to remind ourselves that it is a process within which clinical decisions are made by practitioners, using the best available research evidence, their clinical expertise, and patient preferences, with consideration also of available resources. Stetler, who's model is detailed in Book 1 of this series, and colleagues from the USA (Stetler et al., 1998) suggest that EBP occurs when, within the organization institutionalization of research findings and other objective systematically obtained information has been achieved through the development of culture, capacity and infrastructure. They further argue that this institutionalization of research enhances the practice of clinicians, managers, educators and other staff.

In the subsequent years, in almost all developed, and some developing, countries, healthcare has increased in complexity. For evidence to be successfully implemented into practice, it is essential that the wider issues that can be classed as contextual elements are considered. Such elements are, in general, pertinent to the setting in which the practice change is being proposed and can include leadership; policy; organizational structure, societal, and cultural issues; and basic organizational components. Some of these interact with others, and yet all present different challenges, or influences, to those who are working to get evidence implemented into practice. As a result, it is important that contextual factors are explored in relation to the different healthcare settings that exist worldwide.

It is evident from the literature, and from expert groups, that context can be interpreted in different ways and at different levels. In a concept analysis of context that was introduced in the previous chapter, McCormack et al. (2002) focused primarily on context in terms of environment. By this, they meant the setting where practice takes place, or the setting for the proposed practice change. As the reader will know, there are few environments, if any, that are the same, even within the same area of practice. For example, in the field of critical care, one intensive care unit will have a different environment or be influenced by different environmental factors to that of another unit. The size of the unit, types of patients admitted (e.g., general or specialist), type of organization (public or private), country or geographical location, and the age of the unit; each one of these imposes different influences in unique ways. If these were not enough, there are also the human factors that make one setting different to another. These are often defined as creating the culture of the workplace and this influences the way things are done (Manley, 2000a). Whether context per se is a more significant issue than workplace culture is an issue that is debated in the literature. Davies and colleagues (Davies et al., 2000) for example argue that the key significant factor in the successful uptake of evidence is that of organizational culture and would consider this to be of much greater significance than the issue of context. This conceptualization challenges the perspective offered in models, for example, the Promoting Action on Research Implementation in Health Services (PARIHS) framework where culture is considered to be a sub-element of context. Whatever the answer, the reality is that we know there is an interrelationship between organizational systems, structures, and processes, practice setting and workplace cultures. However, the nature of that relationship (or relationships) remains poorly understood (Plsek & Greenhalgh, 2001).

Berwick, in his work exploring practice change driven by adverse events, has identified the importance of culture (Berwick, 2003). He has been an advocate for practice change for many years now and as head of the US Institute for Health Innovations, he has persuaded hundreds of organizations, and thousands of individuals to adopt evidence-based changes to practice that have positively impacted on many more people's lives. The Institute for Healthcare Improvement (IHI) established a campaign called the 5 million lives campaign that has, at its heart, culture change; for more information on this campaign go to the following web site http://www.ihi.org/IHI/Programs/Campaign (accessed September 28, 2009).

Culture in itself is a major influencing factor on evidence-based practice and on the quest to ensure evidence is translated into practice. This is generally known as knowledge translation. The factors influencing knowledge translation can be further divided by level into micro, meso, and macro. One way of explaining the differences between each of these is to use the work of Kapiriri et al. (2007).

They investigated priority setting at the three different levels in Canada, Norway, and Uganda. They found that at the macro-level, the contextual influences relating to resource allocation decisions were politics, public pressure, and advocacy, some of which were further complicated by the impact of international priorities. At the meso-level, the influencing factors were national priorities, guidelines, and evidence. At the micro-level, however, the contextual influences were much more localized and included attitudes and feelings of worth. Factors that were considered to be at macro-level influenced, or set the context, at the lower meso- and micro-levels.

There are other examples of studies that have been undertaken, which have identified factors that should be considered in terms of care delivery and patient outcomes. Pinkerton and Rivers (2001) explored staffing levels and patient outcomes and identified a number of contextual factors that could also be seen as operating at micro-, meso- and macro-levels. There were factors that could be located at interdepartmental, intradepartmental, the care environment, and external environment levels as well as those that reflected professional competency. The complexity of the relationship between staffing and patient outcomes was acknowledged and further factors identified for consideration: physical environment, organizational culture, operational structure, technology, and support systems. These matched closely those identified in the PARIHS framework: context, culture, leadership, and evaluation (Rycroft-Malone et al., 2002). These five categories of contextual factors were used by Porter-O'Grady and Malloch (2006, p. 204) to reflect possible measurement variables that are associated with these contextual factors and adverse events. We have modified these slightly to help consider factors that might affect evidence implementation in different clinical settings.

- *Physical environment*—number of beds/single rooms; ward layout; noise; meeting rooms
- *Organizational culture*—leadership styles; interdisciplinary communication; values and beliefs
- *Operational structures*—decision-making processes; expertise available; staffing levels; involvement of users in change processes
- *Technology*—information technology availability; level of utilization of computers and electronic decision aids; skills and knowledge of key stakeholders
- *Support systems*—resources; ease of access to a range of support personnel; style of support offered; peer communication; facilitation methods/processes/people.

Models and frameworks

Models or conceptual frameworks can be very useful for facilitating practice change as they identify the concepts or factors that should be considered prior to or during the evidence implementation process. There are a number of pertinent practice change or evidence implementation models, as captured in Book 1 in this series (Rycroft-Malone & Bucknall, eds). Few make explicit how to identify and assess contextual factors. This possibly reflects, as McCormack et al. (2002) point out, the lack of research exploring the impact of context on practice outcomes (p. 264).

Different theoretical explanations of context have been formulated, ranging from artificial intelligence (Franklin, 2003) to Sticht's functional context approach (Sticht, 1975, 1976, 1988). The latter theory is associated with learning and highlights the importance of making learning relevant to the experience of learners and their work context. This association or direction is also applicable to evidence-based practice. Context and the factors associated with this relatively abstract concept can be explored and applied to help make evidence relevant to clinicians as they make decisions in their workplace or as part of their practice.

The principles of the functional context approach listed by Sticht (1975, 1976, 1988) are as follows:

(1) Instruction should be made as meaningful as possible to the learner in terms of the learner's prior knowledge.
(2) Use material and equipment that the learner will actually use after training.
(3) Literacy can be improved by improving content knowledge, information processing skills, or the design of the learning materials.
(4) Valid assessment of learning requires context-/content-specific measurement.

Now applying this to healthcare practice, it is clear that the contextual influences to utilizing evidence in practice need to be made explicit and as meaningful as possible. Therefore it is important that different practice settings consider the contextual factors that are appropriate or relevant to them. Any materials that are used when considering the implementation of evidence into practice need to be contextually relevant and useful, otherwise clinicians will not use them. Finally evaluation of the contextual factors of relevance to a particular setting needs to occur using specific measures, but also needs to reflect the complexity of practice context.

PARIHS

In the 1990s, Kitson and colleagues from the Royal College of Nursing Institute in the UK developed a framework (The PARIHS framework) to guide the implementation of evidence into practice. The full name of the PARIHS framework is the Promoting Action on Research Implementation in Health Services Framework (Kitson et al., 1998; Rycroft-Malone et al., 2002). Three key components were identified (evidence, context, and facilitation) that were inter-related, with implementation being the function of this relationship. McCormack et al. (2002) then used concept analysis techniques to identify the "meaning, characteristic and consequences of practice contexts" (p. 95). The PARIHS framework reflects diagrammatically the interplay between key factors that play a role in the successful implementation of evidence into practice (Rycroft-Malone, 2004). The key components of the context element of the framework are summarized in Table 2.1. Each of these elements has characteristics spanning a continuum of weak to strong. Kitson et al. (1998) proposes that for successful implementation, the evidence needs to be robust, the context needs to be receptive to change, and appropriate facilitation needs to be used.

Although there is still no consensus with regard to defining context, its complexity is acknowledged (McCormack et al., 2002). It is almost impossible to capture all the different contextual factors related to healthcare practice because of the variety of settings, communities, and cultures where healthcare is delivered (p. 96). The environment in healthcare is rarely straightforward but is constantly changing, with many diverse cultures operating at different levels throughout an organization. Research is seen as providing evidence of what might be achieved under ideal circumstances—it creates "context-free" guidance. Of course it is recognized that we do not work in context-free situations, as supported by the Canadian Health Service Research Foundation (CHSRF, 2005, p. 11) who argue that getting evidence into practice is not context free and state: "the role of science is somewhat detached from, and unconcerned with, it's application to specific circumstances." This means that researchers need to consider the context within which the research is being

Table 2.1 Characteristics of the context framework in PARIHS

Elements	Weak characteristics	Strong characteristics
Context	Lack of clarity around boundaries	Boundaries clearly defined (physical, social, cultural, and structural)
	Lack of appropriateness and transparency	Appropriate and transparent decision-making processes
	Lack of information and feedback	Information and feedback
	Lack of power and authority	Power and authority understood
	Not receptive to change	Receptiveness to change
Culture	Unclear values and beliefs	Able to define culture(s) in terms of prevailing values and beliefs
	Low regard for individuals	Values individual staff and clients
	Task-driven organization	Promotes learning organization
	Lack of consistency	Consistency of individual's role or experience to value: relationship with others, team working, power, and authority, rewards/recognition
Leadership	Traditional, command and control leadership	Transformational leadership
	Lack of role clarity	Role clarity
	Lack of teamwork	Effective teamwork
	Didactic approaches to teaching/learning/managing	Enabling/empowering approach to teaching/learning/managing
	Autocratic decision-making processes	Enabling/empowering approach to learning/teaching/managing
Evaluation	Absence of any form of feedback and information	Feedback on individual, team, and systems
	Narrow use of performance information sources	Use of multiple sources of information on performance
	Evaluations rely on single rather than multiple methods	Use of multiple methods (clinical, performance, and experience)
	Poor organizational structure	Effective organizational structure

Source: From McCormack et al. (2008). Reprinted with permission.

undertaken and the effect the context will have when that evidence is put into practice. Moreover, the role of context in the research process needs to be further elucidated (McCormack et al., 2002).

The difficulty in defining and capturing the concept of context has been likened to "trying to catch a cloud" (CHSRF, 2005, p. 13). Context can be seen as "infinite" because it exists in all workplace communities and cultures that are influenced by economic, social, political, fiscal, historical, and psychosocial factors (McCormack et al., 2002). From a review of the relevant literature on context, the Canadian Health Services Research Foundation suggested that issues directly relevant to healthcare include values, political judgments, resources, professional experience and expertise, habits and traditions, lobbyists and pressure groups, and pragmatics and contingencies (CHSRF, 2005). McCormack and colleagues (2002) identified three elements of practice context that need to be assessed in order for research evidence to be utilized—the existing measures of effectiveness, leadership, and culture. Because of the diverse elements of context, it could be concluded that multiple methods of achieving evidence-based practice are needed (Swinburn et al., 2005). However, the framework that emerged from the work of Kitson and colleagues includes three key characteristics of context: culture, leadership, and measurement/evaluation (Rycroft-Malone, 2004).

Culture

Organizational research studies have mainly focused on structure, systems, and behavior (Manley, 2000a,b). Van den Berg and Wilderom (2004) describe organizational culture as the "glue" that holds an organization together and stimulates an employee's commitment to the organization to perform; they suggest that evidence of how to operationalize this "glue" is rare. Davies and colleagues (2000) suggest that, in terms of practice or organizational change, the pertinent aspects of culture associated with a particular organization need to be unpacked. The reason for this is that culture influences the way things are carried out, understood, judged, and valued (Davies et al., 2000, p. 112). They went further to suggest that the elements of culture vary in terms of visibility or consciousness; from unconscious beliefs to those that have great visibility such as ceremonies or traditions that help identify one organization from another. An example of this would be uniforms that bear an organization's logo. Corporate identity is a big business and a great deal of time, effort, and cost are expended in the quest to create an identity that makes the organization stand out or be easily recognized. Schein (1992) believed that the three levels of organizational culture—artifacts, espoused values, and basic assumptions—form a hierarchy. Artifacts are things that are easily seen, highly visible but in many cases can be difficult to understand. Espoused values are conscious strategies, goals, and philosophies. Basic assumptions are the unconscious, taken-for-granted beliefs that may be key to why things do or don't happen. Consequently it is really important to understand the culture of a healthcare setting.

However, Manley (2000a,b) argued that as a concept, organizational culture has little significance to clinicians and patients because of its focus on high-level structures, systems, and processes. Manley showed that individual workplaces have their own cultural characteristics which may be influenced by organizational culture but are unique to each practice setting (i.e., context). These unique characteristics have the greatest influence on the perceptions and experiences of patients and staff about their organization (i.e., workplace culture). Manley (2000a) considered culture in her work evaluating the outcomes of consultant nurses in England and proposed that, at the individual, team, and organizational levels, culture is the driving force shaping the context of the healthcare setting. Schein (1992) considers that organizational culture is the shared value system that builds over time and is used by those within and external to the organization for problem-solving, adapt to changing situations, and work with others.

Manley (2004) defines an ideal culture as "transformational" because it is always changing form, adapting, and responding to a changing context. A transformational culture is based on values that enable staff at all levels to feel empowered, to develop their own potential, and to be innovative in developing practice and thus produce best practice for patients. Manley (2000b) also states that there is a need for qualitative studies to observe the cultures of workplaces and to provide information on how to successfully implement innovative work in practice.

Leadership

Much has been written about what makes a good leader, but the field of nursing has had some difficulty in establishing good leadership (Cunningham, 1998; Girvin, 1998). The most effective leaders are "transformational" ones, who are committed to allowing themselves and others to optimize their skills, abilities, knowledge, and potential (Manley & Dewing, 2002). Leaders described as "transformational" can bring different types of evidence together (research, patient experience, and clinical experience) and implement that evidence into practice, so bringing about new ways of working. In this way they can change the organization's culture and create a context into which evidence-based practice can be more easily integrated

(McCormack et al., 2002). The PARIHS framework points out that everyone can be a leader of something, and that the potential for leadership needs to be developed and released (Rycroft-Malone et al., 2004).

There appear to be elements of leadership that increase the likelihood of success in evidence implementation. These are transformational approach, role clarity, effective teamwork, effective organizational structures, democratic decision-making processes, and when an enabling or empowering approach is evident in the areas of teaching, learning, and managing (McCormack et al., 2002, p. 99). However, it is difficult to objectively determine how these elements relate to each other and if one is more influential than another. A group of knowledge translation researchers (Meijers et al., 2006) explored the literature reporting relationships between context and research utilization by nurses. They suggested that more work is needed before we fully understand the impact of contextual factors on nurses' use of knowledge in their practice.

Evaluation

Evaluating practice takes many forms, from the use of "hard" data (such as cost-effectiveness and length of stay) to "soft" data (such as the patients' experience of practice). In an effective culture, healthcare professionals use evidence gathered from various sources to make decisions about individual or organizational effectiveness; this in turn is used as an integral part of accountability frameworks and staff appraisal strategies (McCormack et al., 2002). This culture embraces peer review, user-led feedback, and reflection on practice, as well as evidence from systematic literature reviews, meta-analyses, and audits of effectiveness. Measurement is a vital part of any environment that seeks to implement evidence into practice—no matter how complex that measurement can be (McCormack et al., 2002).

Despite all of this conceptual level work, the challenge continues to be the identification of the contextual factors that hinder or enhance the implementation of evidence into practice. McCormack et al. (2002) used the concept analysis to refine the factors that appeared, from the literature, to positively or negatively influence the outcome of evidence implementation. Success was deemed to be more likely when the dominant values and beliefs within the organization or setting could be identified and defined, when it is clear that individual staff and clients are valued, if the organization could be classified as a "learning" organization, and when there is consistent teamwork and leadership.

They were able to identify more specific contextual factors that add further to the elements identified in the PARIHS framework. Under the heading of organizational context, access appears to play a significant role in evidence use. In the first place, nurses need to have access to research findings and this may be electronic or via other media. Then they need time to read and appraise the evidence; the latter is associated with knowledge and skills so access to training programs where they can learn about the interpretation and implementation of research findings was considered important (Meijers et al., 2006). Access in terms of human resources featured in the literature reflected the need to have access to knowledge brokers who understand research and practice change. Culture mapped with roles, climate, and support; support was also identified as part of leadership which also mapped with time and education. The PARIHS framework also informed the exploration of context by researchers in Australia (Ellis et al., 2005). They further reiterated the influence that contextual factors impose on settings where practice change was planned.

Context Assessment Index

The Context Assessment Index (CAI) has been developed to provide clinicians with the means to assess and understand the context in which they work and the effect this has on using evidence in practice (McCormack et al., 2009). It consists of a 37-item model, based on the PARIHS theoretical framework. Five factors, collaborative practice, evidence-informed practice, respect for persons, practice boundaries, and evaluation, explained 64% of the variance. The index has been tested and early indications are that it is both reliable and valid. For those who would like the technical data, measures of homogeneity were calculated for each of the five factors; the Cronbach's alpha score for the complete questionnaire was estimated at 0.93, while all five factors achieved a satisfactory estimated level of internal consistency in scoring, ranging from 0.78 to 0.91. Test–retest scores indicate reliability of the findings, and the feedback from focus group participants suggests that the instrument has practical utility.

More recently, McCormack and Wright (2009) undertook a study to test out the usability of the CAI as an instrument for facilitating consciousness rising about the need to develop practice. The CAI was used as a diagnostic tool to determine different clinical settings' "readiness for change" and to develop person-centered continence practice. The CAI highlighted the contextual hurdles (such as task-based care and autocratic leadership) and enabling factors (such as openness to change and transformational leadership) facing the practitioner and the researchers. Understanding these contextual factors is important if we are to develop practice (Scott-Finley & Estabrookes, 2006) and led to different practice development activity based on the contextual hurdles and enablers identified for each site. For example, some areas undertook observations of practice to enhance the understanding of practice context whilst other sites did not need to engage in this activity. The data suggested that the context was so weak in some settings that developing practice was not achievable; for example, one setting had a strong autocratic leader that negatively influenced any progress with change. Through using the CAI, individual team members and whole teams became more aware of the contextual hurdles that were affecting their practice, and preventing initiatives being implemented and sustained in the setting. The CAI is of value in identifying the "readiness" for change and thus the approaches needed for developing practice.

Consistent with the PARIHS framework, facilitation was a key factor to the practitioners' understanding of practice context. Kitson et al. (2008) state facilitation is more effective following a diagnosis of the context. This proved to be of value in the study as once the "context score" was determined, perceptions of context became a focus of discussion, and the congruency (or not) between the outcome of the CAI and the evidence available explored. The process of completing the CAI raised the participants' insights into practice issues. However, without the supporting development work and critical dialogue between participants and a facilitator, insights into practice would have been more limited and change would not have occurred. The teams had the opportunity to discuss and explore practice issues, and facilitation was essential to enable this process. A key factor in the success of the evidence implementation work in each site was the style of leadership. Those sites with transformational leadership achieved the most practice change. In sites that did not have such leadership, the practitioners were lost and frustrated. Individual practitioners were aware of the development issues in their area shown by the feedback received, but due to the leadership of the area felt unable to take this forward. Cultural change cannot come from one person but rather it is a collective process needing all the team on board at different levels (Kitson et al., 2008). For those practitioners who could see what needed to happen to improve practice yet were unable make any impact, they were unable to reach their potential (McCormack & Titchen, 2006).

This small study has shown the value of the CAI as a diagnostic and evaluation tool for understanding practice context and deciding on the appropriate practice development activities to be undertaken. In line with the PARIHS framework, understanding the context was not enough in itself to develop practice, skilled facilitation, and access to appropriate evidence were essential.

The Ottawa Model of Research Use

Another model that has been developed to guide evidence implementation and use is the Ottawa Model of Research Use (OMRU). This was conceptualized by Logan and Graham (Graham & Logan, 2004; Logan & Graham, 1998) and it has been used in a variety of clinical practice settings (Logan et al., 1999; Stacey et al., 2006). The model has gone through some revisions and now includes six key elements:

(1) evidence-based innovation
(2) potential adopters
(3) the practice environment
(4) implementation of interventions
(5) adoption of the innovation
(6) outcomes resulting from implementation of the innovation.

The relationships among the six elements are shown in Figure 2.1. This figure also shows some of the contextual elements that need to be considered as part of the evidence implementation process.

In terms of context, Logan and Graham (Graham & Logan, 2003) stress that the practice environment must be assessed prior to any implementation project commencing. They identified some of the contextual factors that they think should be included in this assessment, and categorized them, as identified in Figure 2.1, under the headings structural, and culture/social. We have listed their suggestions in Table 2.2.

Clinicians in practice settings can use these as prompts to help them understand the factors that might impact on the planned practice

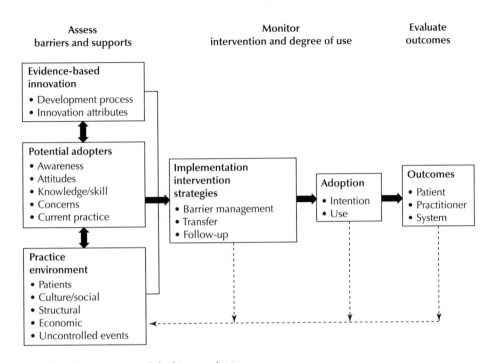

Figure 2.1 The Ottawa Model of Research Use.
Source: Logan et al. (1999). Reproduced with permission from *Canadian Journal of Nursing Research*.

Table 2.2 Assessing structural and cultural contextual factors

Structural factors	Culture/social factors
Decision making	Culture and belief systems
Policies, rules, laws	Leadership
Available technology	Politics and personalities
Physical layout	Patients/consumers
Availability of evidence	Peer influence
Work pressure	
Economic issues	

Source: Adapted from Graham and Logan (2003).

change; an example of the model's use in acute care is provided by Graham and Logan (2004), when they describe the implementation of a skin care clinical practice guideline in Canada. The assessment helped them identify the key barriers within the clinical setting and successfully implement the guideline to enhance the quality of care. Another example focuses on the introduction of an evidence-based family assessment tool within the neonatal intensive care unit environment (Hogan & Logan, 2004). This time the model was used to improve the performance of the neonatal transport team by providing the team with a tool that they could use to assess family responses to the impending transfer of their sick baby to the intensive care unit. This model has proven versatility and as its use increases, more context-specific information will be made available to inform future implementation projects.

Research and development in the field of knowledge translation or evidence implementation continues to occur, building on the work of the researchers such as Graham, Kitson, Rycroft-Malone, McCormack, Stetler, Titler, and others. Book 1 in this series explores the models and theories in more detail, and so these authors' works will not be expanded upon here. Recently, the need to assess social, cultural, and material or environmental contexts was further reinforced by Kontos and Poland (2009). They argue that the existing models, such as Ottawa and PARIHS, albeit very useful, don't include details about how and why the contextual factors interact and how these mechanisms influence knowledge translation. These authors propose a new model to help address some of these limitations, called The Critical Realism and the Arts Utilization Model (CRARUM) and they believe that this has the potential to address the complexities of practice settings, as well as encourage users to engage in critical reflection about the practice change.

Recognition of the complexities of practice settings has not only influenced model development but also led to changes in the ways that knowledge is produced. One such change is explored next, albeit briefly.

Mode 2 thinking and context for evidence-based practice

It is important to keep up-to-date with developments that are taking place in the dynamic area of evidence-based practice. One approach that is beginning to grow in popularity in terms of knowledge generation and implementation is known as Mode 2 thinking. Hessels and Van Lente (2008) suggested that Mode 2 supplemented that of Mode 1 and to help illustrate this, summarized the attributes for each mode (see Table 2.3).

So in relation to the focus of this book, we need to consider Mode 2 knowledge production in terms of its characteristics and how they might be used to assist with clinical decision making and evidence use in practice. Gibbons helps us in this quest (2008) when he linked Mode 2 thinking with knowledge translation at a conference in 2008. The main points that he made have been outlined below.

The first point to note is that Mode 2 knowledge arises directly from the context in which it is needed to be applied or considered. The context of application, therefore, captures all the factors within the environment in which scientific or clinical problems arise, and from this, ways of investigating those problems are developed, the findings or outcomes from the study are disseminated, particularly in terms of who the findings apply or relate to. In other words, who should use this evidence in their practice is defined.

Another characteristic that differentiates Mode 2 from Mode 1 is that it usually involves more than one discipline. This may be in terms of investigators, the range of theories that underpin the work, the sites involved, or the practical approaches that can be used to solve problems. It is more dynamic than Mode 1 and can be responsive to the changing environment; however this makes it more heterogeneous than Mode 1 and so less easy to identify causal factors.

In terms of the context of application, within this approach to knowledge production, it is necessary to reach beyond the knowable context of application to the unknowable context of implication. Here knowledge producers have to reach out and anticipate reflexively the implications of research processes.

As Bamberger suggested, in 2008, the increasing focus on context is helping to blur the division between "micro" and "macro" work.

Table 2.3 Attributes of Mode 1 and Mode 2 knowledge production

Mode 1	Mode 2
Academic context	Context of application
Disciplinary	Transdisciplinary
Homogeneity	Heterogeneity
Autonomy	Reflexivity/social accountability
Traditional quality control (peer review)	Novel quality control

Source: From Hessels and Van Lente (2008, p. 741). Reprinted with permission.

This is creating more robust theories and leading to the exploration of context in diverse settings. Hitt et al. (2007) suggest that exploring phenomena at different levels, rather than just focusing on the micro- or macro-level, better capture the increasing complexity of organizational problems or issues, offering greater predictive power and real-world relevance.

Interestingly the concept of "relevance" has been suggested as being very relevant when considering context, in either theoretical or practical terms (Van Dijk, 1999). Although he suggested this 10 years ago, clearly contextualization has continued to gain prominence when studying issues that reflect or influence social situations. Studies of discourse or communication found that contexts, as well as their instances of text or talk, are unique in that they are never exactly the same. Depending on culture and social situation, factors that might be different include time, place, or circumstances, as well as age, gender, social role, status, beliefs, or aims of participants.

Global factors

Although for many health professionals, the local or national contextual influences have dominance when implementing evidence into practice, we should not lose sight of the wider influence of global contextual factors on evidence use and population health or illness. Wallin (2008) captures this very effectively in an editorial that he wrote in which he drew attention to the high mortality rates among neonates worldwide: "Almost all (99%) neonatal deaths occur in low and middle income countries" (p. 167). As a result of research being carried out in Vietnam, his team has been able to identify some key factors that impact on the success of evidence implementation activities in developing countries. These include underreporting, in this case of mortality, leading to lack of awareness of the extent of the problem, indifference from health professionals and authorities, language, cultural barriers, geographical, and transportation factors.

In many parts of the world, governments acknowledge the importance of evidence-based practice by including the concept in strategic aims and objectives for health. This has been called or labeled as an "adoption in principle," and may be promoted at the national level by the actions of specific advocacy and lobby groups, or the concerted efforts of opinion leaders (Tansella & Thornicroft, 2009).

According to Tansella and Thornicroft, there are two further stages associated with evidence implementation—early implementation and persistence of implementation. These specifically focus on behavior change needed to get evidence practice and then activities aimed at sustaining that change. There are a number of factors that inhibit or encourage this uptake of evidence and these have been summarized in Figure 2.2.

Therefore we have shown, in this chapter, that evidence-based practice requires an active process to take place, to give knowledge translation the best chance of sustained success. It is necessary that the knowledge is contextualized, or adapted, so that it fits with the new setting. There are now tools such as the framework produced by the ADAPTE Collaboration for guideline adaptation. For more information on this, please see http://www.adapte.org/rubrique/the-adapte-collaboration.php (accessed August 10, 2009).

Conclusion

Various models and frameworks help clinicians to understand the contextual factors that may play important roles in the implementation of evidence/knowledge into practice. Context has been called "the sensitizing agent" that increases our awareness of potential influencing factors that might negatively or positively impact on the outcome of the evidence transfer (Bamberger, 2008, p. 840). When these are reviewed it is clear that there are a number of key elements of context that appear to be of greater importance than others, especially when addressing knowledge translation or evidence implementation in healthcare settings. The global financial crisis affecting the world in 2009 highlighted the influence of macro-factors on successful evidence implementation. Whilst guidelines and other forms of evidence can be implemented locally, the sustained effect comes from large-scale strategies, but these are costly. In Australia, the Hand Hygiene Initiative is one example of this. A national approach to tackling shortcoming in hand hygiene practice was launched in 2009, based on the World Health Organization's program, Clean care is safer care, launched in 2005; this was relaunched in 2009 under the campaign named "Save lives; clean your hands." For more information in this initiative in Australia, access the web site: http://www.hha.org.au/home.aspx (accessed November 02, 2009). This site has many resources available for healthcare professionals and consumers to use.

Facilitator/ barrier factors	Level	Phase		
		Adoption: intention to implement EBP	Early implementation of EBP	Persistence of implementation of EBP
	National	Advocacy and lobby groups Policy measures promoting EBP Opinion leaders and champions National policy on financial incentives	Networks of implementation sites Guideline flexibility Guideline feasibility Creation of financial and other incentives Creation of effective monitoring and feedback systems	Networks of implementation sites Consistency and persistence of policy and practice guidance, and financial incentives Effective feedback systems to policy makers
	Local	Local commissioning priorities Opinion leaders and champions Clinical and professional culture	Initial availability of resources to implement EBP Information technology systems Leadership and champions Consistency of local policy and practice guidance Clinical and professional culture Staff financial and other incentives Training Systems for assessing practice fidelity	Continuing availability of resources to implement EBP Staff turnover and continuing staff training Clinical and professional culture Financial and other staff incentives Systems to assess practice fidelity Effective feedback systems to staff
	Individual	Patient advocacy Carer advocacy Practitioner preferences	Practitioner preferences and characteristics Academic detailing Knowledge/training about EBP Awareness of litigation about EBP Patient characteristics and preferences	Academic detailing Awareness of litigation about EBP

Each of the factors described may act as either a facilitator or a barrier. The grey elements represent potential gaps or barriers between the three stages and the three levels of implementation.

Figure 2.2 Facilitators and barriers to the implementation of evidence-based practice (EBP).
Source: From Tansella and Thornicroft (2009). Reproduced with permission from *British Journal of Psychiatry.*

Hitt et al. (2007) suggested that, rather than categorizing contextual factors by micro-, meso- and macro-levels, it may be more effective to consider factors at different levels. Work pressures would be one contextual factor that is highly pertinent to assess in today's complex world. Globally, nursing shortages appear to pose challenges to those facilitating or leading practice changes across the world, as the multinational workforce brings with it variations in practice, attitudes, beliefs, and societal norms. At the more local level, organizations that employ higher proportions of temporary staff, or where turnover is high, appear to offer lower quality care reflected in higher levels of adverse events (Stanton & Rutherford, 2004).

Another contextual factor that should be considered by all evidence implementers is that of information technology. The availability of computers to source evidence, and to guide decision making in practice cannot be assumed. Where there are few resources, it is harder for healthcare professionals to access up-to-date information and utilize this to inform their practice. Each of the models includes this as a potential barrier and this should continue to be the case for the foreseeable future.

The involvement of patients, clients, or service users in the implementation of evidence is something that we should be actively encouraging and exploring new ways of working or research designs that incorporate user views. The work of Kontos and Poland (2009) offers potential for knowledge generation in relation to this. Clients' views have been explicitly included as a key source of knowledge or evidence in the definitions of evidence-based practice and it is important that these are assessed as contextual factors that might inhibit or enable evidence implementation.

The limitations of traditional forms of evidence or knowledge generation have generated significant debate; we contributed to this by including the discussion on Mode 2 thinking. Recently the debate was moved forward in an article published in *Implementation Science*; Leykum and colleagues (2009) highlight the challenges generated from the desire to utilize multipronged interventions that increase the likelihood of successful implementation of evidence, and the complexities of practice settings that make effective translation of the evidence really difficult due to local contextual factors. They addressed this by proposing the adoption of a mixed method approach that combined participatory action research (PAR) with randomized controlled trial (RCT) design. This, they believe, would be a win–win since the rigor of the RCT would be complemented by the collaborative, cyclical, reflective qualities embedded within PAR. This would require a less-prescriptive approach than usually associated with RCTs and have locally designed interventions that address a common goal. They suggest that this combination, specifically the PAR, will be more effective in meeting the goals of implementation research, achieving generalizability, and accommodating local contextual factors that are associated with complex, dynamic healthcare settings or organizations. We need to pay close attention to this debate and the new strategies that are being proposed to overcome the limitations associated with traditional implementation research. Designing studies that are conceptually informed by models or tools that include contextual factors inevitably encapsulates the need for locally developed interventions; the key is to identify the common factors and also to understand more fully the mechanisms of interaction between these factors. These endeavors will keep those involved in evidence implementation busy for several years to come.

In the following chapters, readers will see how experts working in various clinical settings assess and interpret the contextual elements outlined in this chapter, and apply that knowledge as part of the evidence implementation process.

References

Bamberger, P. (2008). Beyond conceptualization: Using context theories to narrow the micro–macro gap in management research. *Academy of Management Journal*, 51, 839–846.

Berwick, D. (2003). Disseminating innovations in health care. *JAMA*, 289, 1969–1975.

Canadian Health Service Research Foundation (CHSRF) (2005). Conceptualising and combining evidence for health system guidance (final report). Ontario, Canada: Canadian Health Service Research Foundation.

Cunningham, G. (1998). *The RCN Leadership Programme*. London: Royal College of Nursing.

Davies, H.T.O., Nutley, S.M. & Mannion, R. (2000). Organisational culture and quality of health care. *Quality in Health Care*, 9, 111–119.

Ellis, I., Howard, P., Larson, A. & Robertson, J. (2005). From exploration to work practice: An exploration of context and facilitation in the development of evidence-based practice. *Worldviews on Evidence-Based Nursing*, 2, 84–93.

Fineout-Overholt, E., Levin, R.F. & Melnyk, B.M. (2004). Strategies for advancing evidence-based practice in clinical settings. *The Journal of the New York State Nurses' Association*, 35, 28–32.

Franklin, J. (2003). The representation of context: Ideas from artifical intelligence. *Law, Probability and Risk*, 2, 191–199.

Gibbons, M. (2008). Why is knowedge translation important? Grounding the conversation. *Focus*. Available at http://www.ncddr.org/kt/products/focus/focus21/ (accessed May 25, 2009).

Girvin, J. (1998). *Leadership in Nursing (Essentials of Nursing Management)*. London: Palgrave Macmillan.

Graham, I. & Logan, J. (2003). Ottowa model of research use: A pragmatic conceptual model for knowledge translation. *Knowledge Translation ICE Team Meeting*. Ottowa, Canada: KT-ICEBeRG/GReBECI.

Graham, K. & Logan, J. (2004). Using the Ottawa Model of Research Use to implement a skin care program. *Journal of Nursing Care Quality*, 19, 18–24.

Hessels, L. & Van Lente, H. (2008). Re-thinking new knowledge production: A literature review and a research agenda. *Research Policy*, 37, 740–760.

Hitt, M.A., Beamish, P.W., Jackson, S.E. & Mathieu, J. (2007). Building theoretical and empirical bridges across levels: Multilevel research in management. *Academy of Management Journal*, 50, 1385–1399.

Hogan, D. & Logan, J. (2004). The Ottawa Model of Research Use: A guide to clinical innovation in the NICU. *Clinical Nurse Specialist*, 18, 255–261.

Kapiriri, L., Norheim, O.F. & Martin, D.K. (2007). Priority setting at the micro-, meso- and macro-levels in Canada, Norway and Uganda. *Health Policy*, 82, 78–94.

Kitson, A., Harvey, G. and McCormack, B. (1998). Approaches to implementing research in practice. *Quality in Health Care*, 7, 149–159.

Kitson, A.L., Rycroft-Malone, J., Harvey, G., Mccormack, B., Seers, K. & Titchen, A. (2008). Evaluating the successful implementation of evidence into practice using the PARIHS framework: Theoretical and practice challenges. *Implementation Science*, 3, 1.

Kontos, P. & Poland, B. (2009). Mapping new theoretical and methodological terrain for knowledge translation: Contributions from critical realism and the arts. *Implementation Science*, 4, 1.

Leykum, L., Pugh, J., Lanham, H., Harmon, J. & McDaniel, R. (2009). Implementation research design: Integrating participatory action research into randomized controlled trials. *Implementation Science*, 4, 1.

Logan, J. & Graham, I.D. (1998). Toward a comprehensive interdisciplinary model of health care research use. *Science Communication*, 20, 227–246.

Logan, J., Harrison, M.B., Graham, I.D., Dunn, K. & Bissonnette, J. (1999). Evidence-based pressure-ulcer practice: The Ottawa Model of Research Use. *Canadian Journal of Nursing Research*, 31, 37–52.

Manley, K. (2000a). Organisational culture and consultant nurse outcomes: Part 1. Organisational culture. *Nursing Standard*, 14, 34–38.

Manley, K. (2000b). Organisational culture and consultant nurse outcomes: Part 2. Nurse outcomes. *Nursing Standard*, 14, 34–39.

Manley, K. (2004). Transformational culture: A culture of effectiveness. In: McCormack, B., Manley. K. & Garbett, R. (eds) *Practice Development in Nursing*. Oxford: Blackwell.

Manley, K. & Dewing, J. (2002). The consultant nurse role. *NHS Journal of Healthcare Professionals*, Spring, 8–9.

McCormack, B. & Titchen, A. (2006). Critical creativity: Melding, exploding, blending. *Educational Action Research*, 14, 239–266.

McCormack, B. & Wright, J. (2009). Using the Context Assessment Index (CAI) in practice: Facilitating consciousness raising for practice development. Newtownabbey, Co. Antrim: University of Ulster.

McCormack, B., Kitson, A., Harvey, G., Rycroft-Malone, J., Titchen, A. & Seers, K. (2002). Getting evidence into practice: The meaning of "context." *Journal of Advanced Nursing*, 38, 94–104.

McCormack, B., McCarthy, G., Wright, J., Coffey, A. & Slater, P. (2008). *Development of the Context Assessment Index (CAI)*. Belfast, Northern Ireland: University of Ulster & University of Cork.

McCormack, B., McCarthy, G., Wright, J., Coffey, A. & Slater, P. (2009). Development and testing of the Context Assessment Index (CAI). *Worldviews on Evidence-Based Nursing*, 6, 27–35.

Meijers, J.M.M., Janssen, M.A.P., Cummings, G.G., Wallin, L., Estabrooks, C.A. & Halfens, R.Y.G. (2006). Assessing the relationships between contextual factors and research utilization in nursing: Systematic literature review. *Journal of Advanced Nursing*, 55, 622–635.

Pinkerton, S. & Rivers, R. (2001). Integrated delivery systems. Factors influencing staffing needs. *Nursing Economics*, 19, 236.

Plsek, P. & Greenhalgh, T. (2001). Complexity science: The challenge of complexity in health care. *British Medical Journal*, 323, 625–628.

Porter-O'Grady, T. & Malloch, K. (2006). Partnership economics: Creating value through evidence-based workload management. In: Malloch, K. & Porter-O'Grady, T. (eds) *Introduction to Evidence-Based Practice in Nursing and Healthcare*. Sudbury, MA: Jones & Bartlett.

Rycroft-Malone, J. (2004). The PARIHS framework—A framework for guiding the implementation of evidence-based practice. Promoting Action on Research Implementation in Health Services. *Journal of Nursing Care Quality*, 19, 297–304.

Rycroft-Malone, J., Kitson, A., Harvey, G. et al. (2002). Ingredients for change: Revisiting a conceptual framework. *Quality and Safety in Health Care*, 11, 174–180.

Schein, E.H. (1992). *Organizational Culture and Leadership*. San Francisco: Jossey-Bass.

Scott-Finley, S. & Estabrookes, C.A. (2006). Mapping the organisational culture research in nursing: A literature review. *Journal of Advanced Nursing*, 56, 498–513.

Stacey, D., Pomey, M.-P., O'Conner, A.M. & Graham, I.D. (2006). Adoption and sustainability of decision support for patients facing health decisions: An implementation case study in nursing. *Implementation Science*, 1, 17.

Stanton, M. & Rutherford, M. (2004). Hospital nurse staffing and quality of care. *Research in Action*. Rockville: Agency for Healthcare Research and Quality.

Stetler, C.B., Brunell, M., Giuliano, K.K., Morsi, D., Prince, L. & Newell-Stokes, V. (1998). Evidence-based practice and the role of nursing leadership. *Journal of Nursing Administration*, 28, 45–53.

Sticht, T.G. (1975). Applications of the audread model to reading evaluation and instruction. In: Resnick, L. & Weaver, P. (eds) *Theory and Practice of Early Reading*. Hillsdale, NJ: Erlbaum.

Sticht, T.G. (1976). Comprehending reading at work. In: Just, M. & Carpenter, P. (eds) *Cognitive Processes in Comprehension*. Hillsdale, NJ: Erlbaum.

Sticht, T. (1988). *Adult Literacy Education*. Washington, DC: American Education Research Association.

Swinburn, B., Gill, T. & Kumanyika, S. (2005). Obesity prevention: A proposed framework for translating evidence into action. *Obesity Reviews*, 6, 23–33.

Tansella, M. & Thornicroft, G. (2009). Implementation science: Understanding the translation of evidence into practice. *The British Journal of Psychiatry*, 195, 283–285.

Van den Berg, P.T. & Wilderom, C. (2004). Defining, measuring, and comparing organizational cultures. *Applied Psychology: An International Review*, 53, 570–582.

Van Dijk, T.A. (1999). On context. *Discourse & Society*, 10, 291–292.

Wallin, L. (2008). Evidence-based practice in a global context: The case of neonatal mortality. *Worldviews on Evidence-Based Nursing*, 5, 167–169.

Chapter 3

Making context work in primary health care

John Rosenberg and Debbie Kralik

Introduction

Health care in the community setting is one of the more challenging contexts for evidence-based practice. Community-based care comprises more than simply transplanting hospital care into people's homes; in addition to the provision of supportive services, it also takes a range of approaches to health care practice that promotes optimal health and builds the capacity of individuals and communities to respond to their health needs.

Primary health care is comprised of the diverse activities that build sustainable community capacity to achieve health and well-being throughout all of life's stages. The expansive nature of primary health care means that a map for practice is not feasible; however a framework which can be adapted to suit the variety of situations and practice settings can be identified. The focus of this chapter is to broadly define and explore the principles of primary health care and consider the contexts of primary health care in relation to evidence-based practice.

Not to be confused with primary health care, "primary care" refers to the activities of a health care provider who acts as a first point of consultation for patients and as such is an important form of health access in the community setting (Nesbitt & Hanna, 2008). It is the part of the health care system that, in many parts of the world, people interact with most of the time. Continuity of care is a key characteristic of primary care. Primary care involves the widest scope of health care and is inclusive of people across the life span, from all socioeconomic and geographic origins, including those seeking to maintain optimal health, people with multiple chronic diseases, and those at the end of their lives.

Despite these important definitional distinctions, both the published literature and in practice reflect poor understanding of the differences between the two.

What is primary health care?

Primary health care (PHC) was formally recognized as a framework to improve the world's health in 1978 with the *Declaration of Alma Ata*.

Primary health care seeks to extend the first level of the health system from sick care to the development of health. It seeks to protect health and detect problems at an early stage. Primary health care services involve continuity of care, health promotion, and education, integration of prevention with sick care, a concern for population as well as individual health, community involvement, and the use of appropriate technology (WHO, 1978).

The PHC values to achieve health, for all require health systems that put people at the center of health care (WHO, 2007). What people consider desirable ways of living as individuals and what they expect for their communities constitute important parameters for provision of PHC.

Primary health care encompasses diagnosis and therapy, but it has a much broader scope. It includes coordinating, integrating, and expanding systems and services to provide more population health and public health services, not necessarily only those provided by medical doctors. It encourages the best use of all health providers to maximize the potential of all health resources in the system.

So what constitutes a healthy community? The Ontario Health Communities Coalition (ND) suggests that a health community includes the following factors:

- clean and safe physical environment
- peace, equity, and social justice
- adequate access to food, water, shelter, income, work, and leisure activities
- access to health care services
- opportunities for learning and development of skills

- supportive relationships and networks
- workplaces that support family well-being
- processes for residents to participate in decision making
- cultural and spiritual heritage
- diverse and vital economy
- protection of the natural environment
- responsible and sustainable use of resources.

These factors reflect the personal, professional, and community perspectives of community health. When people are healthy, they are able to reach their potential. There is a balance between the barriers to health (such as unemployment) and the factors that encourage health (such as education, sporting facilities). Health in this context is the dynamic relationship between the physical, emotional, social, and spiritual dimensions and the environment. Communities are systems of interactive relationships between people and their physical, geographic, personal, and social networks (McMurray, 2003). This is precisely the context for primary health care.

Drawing on the WHO definition, Rogers and Veale (2000) suggest primary health care can be comprised of three interrelated elements: a philosophy of practice, a set of strategies, and a level of service provision. Nesbitt and Hanna (2008) support these views.

PHC as a philosophy of practice

Primary health care is characterised by a "holistic understanding of health as wellbeing, rather than the absence of disease" (Rogers & Veale, 2000, p. 5). The philosophy of primary health care is built on a holistic understanding and recognition of the multiple (social, economic, environmental, cultural, etc.) determinants of health, equity in health care, community participation, and control over health services, and a focus on health promotion and disease prevention. It includes the concepts of health promotion, population health, and community development.

PHC as a set of strategies

Primary health care involves a "set of strategies aimed at creating health care which is consistent with the underlying philosophy" (Rogers & Veale, 2000). These strategies are based on the following premises: needs-based planning; decentralized management; education; inter-sectoral coordination and cooperation; balance between health promotion, prevention, and treatment; and multidisciplinary health workers.

PHC as a level of service provision

As a level of service provision, primary health care includes service delivery that is in line within the underlying philosophy. Primary health care services are locally based; affordable and accessible; well integrated; and built on health care teams. Primary health care services include health promotion, rehabilitation, disease prevention, and illness treatment; more recently, the provision of end-of-life care has become increasingly understood in a public health context, with a number of services framing their models of care in this way. Perhaps what is most important to remember is that primary health care is applicable for all aspects of health service provision, from acute hospital services to health promotion programs to end-of-life care.

Principles of primary health care

Ideally, primary health care is organized within an integrated team and supported by a community network that includes, as partners, not only the health care workers and service providers but also the community itself. In addition, an approach to health care based on primary health care principles is valid for both acute and community care settings.

A primary health care approach moves beyond the individual and the medical and/or nursing diagnosis (clinical and curative approach) to view the larger social picture of people in the context of socio-economic, cultural, and political environment. The PHC approach considers the way in which the context affects health and then acts upon this information. The principles of PHC give attention to:

- equity
- social determinants of health
- population health approach
- health promotion
- consumer and community participation
- collaborating with others
- working across the continuum of care
- working in teams.

Building on the *Declaration of Alma Ata*, the WHO's *Ottawa Charter for Health Promotion* in 1986 described the components of healthy communities; *building healthy public policy* refers to advocating a clear political commitment to health and equity in all sectors, and the *creation of supportive environments* refers to health promotion that generates living and working conditions that are safe, stimulating, satisfying, and enjoyable. At the heart of the process of *strengthening community action* is the empowerment of communities through developing ownership and control over their endeavors and destinies. Health promotion supports personal and social development through the provision of information and education for health, enhancing health skills, and these activities are coined as *developing personal skills*. This works to increase the options available to people for them to exercise more control over their health. *Reorienting of health services* views the role of the health sector as moving increasingly in a health promotion direction, beyond its responsibility for providing clinical and curative services. The reorienting includes expanding the health service mandate to one that is sensitive and respects diverse cultural needs.

The translation of these broad-reaching and ambitious principles presents many challenges to those working to enhance evidence-based practice in the primary health care setting. For example, as health professionals we see the impact of inequality when health care is not affordable or when access to health services is denied. We can take into account these principles but we may feel that the agenda to change these are beyond the scope in our everyday practice. This we need to engage more actively in discussion of the challenges facing primary health care practitioners.

What are the challenges?

Historically, primary care has tended to represent the traditional medical model of response to illness and associated responsibilities. The associated lack of a person-centered focus from health care services meant that care people experienced was fragmented, poorly informed in terms of their individual care needs and options, and that there were gaps and/or duplication of services received. These factors can be compounded by underdeveloped self-care skills, low levels of health literacy, a lack of available and reliable information, and limited health practitioner support. Overall, this approach can lead to reduced adherence to treatment regimes, limited success with reduction in lifestyle-related risk factors and worsening clinical outcomes. This is demonstrated in the following example from the author's practice.

Jim is aged in his forties and has had asthma for several years with related breathing difficulties. Jim sees a GP when he is feeling unwell and has presented to Emergency Departments on several occasions when he has had acute asthma. His GP provided a generic asthma management plan for Jim at a previous visit but he has not been able to make the changes needed to incorporate the treatment regime into his daily life, and does not use asthma preventer and reliever medications as directed, or regularly enough. Jim has been a heavy smoker most of his adult life and though he has reduced the amount he smokes, he continues to smoke. Although advised to quit smoking, exercise more and lose weight, Jim is yet to take up this advice and may need better support and information to help him change his lifestyle.

Jim does not have a clear understanding of his condition and what sorts of things are likely to provoke an asthma attack. The treatment and advice he has received to date has tended to focus on the problem of his asthma, not on Jim's overall health needs as a person, including what he needs to manage his asthma, and how to address the barriers that are preventing him from making lifestyle changes.

Primary health care providers in today's world need to work with people to develop capacity to take responsibility for their own care and to facilitate independence rather than create dependence. This represents a major shift in thinking and a change in approach for many health professionals. Initiatives focusing on self-care have been taking place in Scotland for several years now and the work is beginning to impact positively on health outcomes for those with chronic diseases such as heart failure and chronic obstructive pulmonary diseases—for more information see the Alliance for Self Care Research at their web site: http://www.ascr.ac.uk/.

There are a number of patient and provider issues in the primary health care system, including:

- the fragmentation of care and services
- the lack of emphasis on health
- barriers to access
- the need for public education and awareness
- poor information sharing, collection, and management.

Other widely identified fundamental systemic concerns include:

- the accountability of both patients and providers
- the unequal distribution of resources
- the misalignment of incentives, especially fee-for service remuneration that rewards episodic care
- systemic inflexibility in situations where support is needed to nurture innovation in approaches or organizational refinement in keeping with local needs and circumstances
- inadequate attention being paid to some providers, especially in rural and remote areas, and to groups such as indigenous Australians.

Research evidence has demonstrated that there are strong links between income and the health status of people (Keating & Hertzman, 1999; Labonte, 2001). Health care needs to be available where people live and work. Often a significant barrier to accessing health care is geographic location, particularly for people living in rural and remote areas (McMurray, 2003). People living in cities can also experience difficulty accessing services but often for different reasons. Therefore, when considering the contextual factors that may positively or negatively impact on practice change associated with the translation of evidence into practice, it is important that macro and micro factors such as these are embraced and acknowledged.

Making context work in primary care

The environmental context of PHC is the community; however, it is imperative to understand that this term does not describe a homogeneous group. "The community" is, of course, as diverse as its members, both individually and collectively. The issue that we need to explore is how to effectively work within the community context. We propose two fundamental strategies to address this complexity: *assessing community need* and *engaging community*.

Assessing community need

Responsiveness to needs is one of the leading PHC principles. It is important to assess the needs of a community so that responsive services can be developed based on need. One important activity for any health professional working in the community is ascertaining need. Here it is argued that health service delivery in all parts of the world should be based on the identified needs of the clients/community. It is necessary for health professionals to formally identify, on a regular basis, the gaps in health care service—and wherever possible, to subsequently adjust service delivery based upon the needs identified pertaining to the service gap. Synonymous with this aim is the identification of what groups of persons are accessing health services in proportion to their representation within the general population of the community served—and to ascertain the reasons for any disparity. In this sense, the term community can be viewed as:

- structure or locale
- the people
- the social systems.

Community assessment is not an end in itself but provides a guide to action. A complete assessment involves a careful look at each component to begin to identify needs for health policy, health program development, health issues, and service provision. These data provide evidence for decision makers within the organizations and in the wider political arena and toward healthy public policy. Wass (2000) proposes that community assessment should be carried out with full participation of community members and that participatory approaches are central to PHC. She defines community assessment as:

> A comprehensive description of needs of a population that is defined or defines itself, as a community, and the resources that exist within that community, carried out with active involvement of the community itself, for the purpose of developing an action plan or other means of improving the quality of life in the community
>
> (Wass, 2000, p. 87)

Three central issues are identified by this definition:

(1) Community assessment is a process of determining both the needs and the resources of a community.
(2) Community assessment could be carried out with the active participation of community members.

(3) Community assessments are carried out for the specific purpose of achieving change that improves the quality of life of those living in the community. *It is a guide to ACTION.*

Wass (2000) details the four ways in which needs can be classified. These include:

(1) *Felt needs*—what people say they need
(2) *Expressed needs*—demonstrated by people's use of services
(3) *Normative needs*—determined on the basis of research
(4) *Comparative needs*—determined by comparing the services available in one geographical area to another geographical area.

It is important to realize that there is no set formula for carrying out a needs assessment. It involves fitting together bits of information to produce a complete picture of the issues.

The skills required for assessing individual clients and those used for assessing community needs are the same: listening and observation. When assessing community needs the following may assist:

- learn about the history of the community
- listening to the community (active listening)
- observe your community (walk, don't drive)
- social and economic indicators (proportion of people in each age group, income levels, number of people on each type of pension, number of single-parent families, number of single-income families, and level of home ownership)
- epidemiological data (distribution and determinants of disease in human populations).

Community assessment should be an integral part of health promotion work, thereby reflecting a social view of health. It should recognize the partnership between people and health workers in determining their needs and services, planning action, and evaluating outcomes (Wass, 2000).

Engaging community

The utilization of primary health care as an approach to the promotion of optimal health in the community context is not simply "just another thing to do" in the busy schedules of community-based health care practitioners. Rather, it provides a "lens" through which the operationalization of health-promoting strategies can be developed, implemented, and evaluated. This perspective is one of "working with" rather than "working for" the community; it is one of engagement, rather than provision. Through this engagement, community-based health care organizations are enabled to be responsive to the needs of the community in which they are present. Using the three elements of community described above (the locale, the people, and the social systems), we examine the central role context plays in the utilization of primary health care.

Example 1—Context determined by the locale

The health challenges faced by rural and remote communities the world over are substantial, where determinants of morbidity and mortality exceed those identified in city populations; rural communities have higher rates of coronary heart disease, pulmonary disease, and other chronic illnesses, as well as higher incidences of motor vehicle accidents and suicide (Baum, 2008; McMurray, 2003). Ironically, even in countries described as "resource rich"—such as USA, Canada, and Australia—rural communities are often under-resourced in the provision of health care services compared to their metropolitan counterparts. Notably, however, members of rural communities describe themselves as living healthier lives than their metropolitan counterparts despite the stressors inherent in rural living (McMurray, 2003). Many rural dwellers would identify a "stronger sense of community" than that found in cities and this may translate into improved relational continuity (Haggerty et al., 2008). Under these circumstances, primary health care may provide an approach to optimizing the health of rural communities.

In Ontario, Canada, the health of the indigenous population has led to the development of an initiative called the Indigenous Health Research Knowledge Transfer/Translation Network (IHRKTN). The development of evidence-based practices and the translation of knowledge that are aligned with the needs of the community, determined by the locale acknowledge and recognize the diverse organizational and cultural environment. The group's strategy aims to "a) improve the two-way flow of relevant and respectful information between Aboriginal health organizations and researchers, b) to evaluate best practices over time and to c) enhance the training and awareness of future researchers about appropriate KT practices."

(Randford & Warry, ND, http://socserv.socsci.mcmaster.ca/ihrktn/ihrkt-images/KTsurveyresults.pdf).

In his examination of the international literature on PHC in rural and remote communities, Wakerman (2009, p. 22) identifies these principles that appear to contribute to the success of PHC organizations:

- the need for adequate funding and appropriate financing mechanisms
- community participation
- health information systems
- multidisciplinary practice
- vision or leadership.

Nevertheless, he cautions that, whilst the uptake of PHC in many communities has been significant in various parts of the world, there is a lack of rigorous evidence regarding the success of these strategies.

The practice of health care by professionals in rural communities has been described as one of "mixed blessings"; as highly visible members of the community, the rural practitioner is usually known, judged, and available around the clock (Francis & Chapman, 2008). However, when implementing PHC approaches, providing leadership to a community of which the health professional is a member can promote community engagement in ways that a purely professional approach might not. Community attachment has been described by Kulig and colleagues (2009) as a key factor in recruitment and retention of the primary health care workforce.

Example 2—Context determined by the people

Whilst not always thought of as a field of health care amenable to primary health care, in the past decade or so, there has been growing interest in the fusion of primary health care/health promotion and end-of-life care (Kellehear, 1999, 2005; Rao et al., 2002, 2005; Rosenberg, 1992; Rosenberg & Yates, 2010a). Palliative care, with its origins in the modern hospice movement, has a strong record of community engagement that has it well placed for this fusion to be undertaken in palliative care services (Rosenberg & Yates, 2010b).

In a recent study in an Australian city, the evaluation of community engagement was undertaken in a community-based home hospice service (Rosenberg, 2007). The hospice's vision statement clearly articulated its intention to work toward:

> ... the creation of a healthy community attitude in relation to death and dying and its mission is to promote hospice philosophy and provide hospice services to the members of our community who are affected by death and dying.

Alongside its provision of clinical palliative care services for those at the end of life, the promotion of community health specifically around issues of death and dying was operationalized through a number of strategies. This included a series of death education programs, targeting the wider public; based upon an assessment that the community was ill-equipped to deal with end-of-life issues, the hospice service developed—with consumer input—a program. Details of the program were distributed amongst community and corporate groups with current program schedules. Its goals were directed at potential participants, and aimed to assist them to (Rosenberg, 2007, pp. 159–160):

- become better equipped to deal with everyday stresses and important issues in their life, teaching the participants how to work with them
- gain insights into the effects personal thoughts have on general happiness, well-being, and their interactions with others
- apply self-awareness in transforming their thoughts using guided visualization, breathing techniques, and different forms of meditation
- establish a daily meditation practice
- strengthen personal capacity to manage physical and/or emotional pain
- develop a greater capacity for happiness and love, for self and others.

This program was founded clearly upon health promotion principle of *strengthening community action*, which we have described here as the empowerment of communities through developing ownership and control over their endeavors and destinies. In this study, this activity was viewed as a key strategy in shifting the focus from service provision to engagement; in the words of this study respondent:

> The wider community needs to be doing something so that ... dying doesn't belong to a hospice service ... it belongs to the community.

(Rosenberg, 2007, p. 222)

Rather than merely shifting responsibility for dealing with end-of-life issues, respondents described a community empowered to articulate their wishes for end-of-life care and their place in the communities to which they belong:

> The community needs to be more involved in saying . . . "Yes, we want palliative care, we want to die at home, we want to be active people until we die, we want to be making a contribution to the community until we die, my family needs to get back into the community after I've died."

To reiterate an earlier point, this practice example illustrates how community assessment:

- is a process of determining both the needs and the resources of a community.
- could be carried out with the active participation of community members.
- is carried out for the specific purpose of achieving change that improves the quality of life of those living in the community.

Example 3—Context determined by the social system

The health care reform and integration of PHC as a fundamental approach to health care in Canada provides one of the best examples of how social and political systems provide a context for the implementation of PHC. In their review of PHC reform, Lamarche et al. (2003) proposed that an *integrated community model* provided the highest quality, most cost-effective and most equitable approach to the provision of health care. Whilst limited in aspects of accessibility and responsiveness, this particular PHC model was recommended as a benchmark for reform of health care in Canada.

Based on community engagement, the integrated community model of primary health care is characterized by the integration of health care services simultaneously with the community and the wider systems of governance in the jurisdiction (Lamarche et al., 2003). It includes the governance of services by consumers, small local centers focussed on health promotion, the provision of continuity of *primary care* by the professional team, and the utilization of information technology and other mechanisms to integrate with the rest of the health care system. Funding for this PHC approach is an integral component of the jurisdiction's government. This model is analogous to the UK's Primary Care Trusts and Scandinavian health care centers.

Conclusion

In this chapter, we have described contexts in primary health care, incorporating components of health promotion, community assessment, and community engagement. The barriers to using evidence in practice in primary care settings have been identified by McKenna et al. in 2004; not surprisingly the issues of accessing evidence, not feeling empowered to implement changes, and difficulties with patient compliance are all factors that affect other settings as you will see as you read the other chapters in this book. However, what we have tried to do here is move beyond these known barriers and focus on the broader, contextual factors that are, in many ways, unique to primary health care settings across the world. The PHC principles can transcend continents and be applied in different countries with differing systems of health care delivery. We can learn a lot from the examples given here, and begin to take on board the messages being conveyed. The needs of the rural and remote populations throughout the world are complex and require tailored approaches; so too in many ways are those in the urban areas where ease of access is often assumed and yet uptake of services can be poor for many different reasons.

For evidence to the embedded into practice, we need to take note of the importance of community assessment. We also need to communicate with each other to ensure that lessons learnt in one setting can be considered by those implementing evidence in another. There are resources available and we need to utilize them; take for example the Primary Health Care Research and Information Service in Australia (http://www.phcris.org.au/). This provides clinicians, researchers, and the community with information about initiatives taking place in order to facilitate generating and managing information about Australian primary health care. Let us consider the common issues, then the contextual factors that affect the setting and, with persistence and drive, ensure that there is optimal uptake of best available evidence into practice.

References

Baum, F. (2008). *The New Public Health*. South Melbourne: Oxford University Press.

Francis, K. & Chapman, Y. (2008). Rural and remote community nursing. In: Kralik, D. & van Loon, A. (eds) *Community Nursing in Australia*. Carlton, Australia: Blackwell Publishing.

Haggerty, J.L., Pineault, R., Beaulieu, M-D. et al. (2008). Practice features associated with patient-reported accessibility, continuity, and coordination of primary health care. *Annals of Family Medicine*, 6(12): 116–123.

Keating, D. & Hertzman, C. (1999). *Developmental Health and Wealth of Nations: Social, Biological and Educational Dynamics*. New York: The Guilford Press.

Kellehear, A. (1999). *Health Promoting Palliative Care*. Oxford: Oxford University Press.

Kellehear, A. (2005). *Compassionate Cities: Public Health and End-of-Life Care*. London: Routledge.

Kulig, J.C., Stewart, N., Penz, K., Forbes, D., Morgan, D. & Emerson, P. (2009). Work setting, community attachment, and satisfaction among rural and remote nurses. *Public Health Nursing*, 26(5), 430–439.

Labonte, R. (2001). Health promotion in the 21st century: Celebrating the ordinary, *Health Promotion Journal of Australia*, 12(2): 104–109.

Lamarche, P.A., Beaulieu, M.-D., Pineault, R., Contandriopoulos, A.-P., Denis, J.-L. & Haggerty, J. (2003). *Choices for Change: The Path for Restructuring Primary Healthcare Services in Canada*. Ottawa, Ontario, Canada: Canadian Health Services Research Foundation, pp. 1–38.

McKenna, H.P., Ashton, S. & Keeney, S. (2004). Barriers to evidence-based practice in primary care. *Journal of Advanced Nursing*, 45(2), 178–189.

McMurray, A. (2003). *Community Health and Wellness: A Socioecological Approach*, 2nd ed. Marrickville, NSW: Elsevier.

Nesbitt, P. & Hanna, B. (2008). Primary health care. In: Kralik, D. & van Loon, A. (eds) *Community Nursing in Australia*. Carlton, Australia: Blackwell Publishing.

Ontario Healthy Communities Coalition (ND). What makes a healthy community? Available at http://www.ohcc-ccso.ca/en/what-makes-a-healthy-community. (accessed November 20, 2009).

Randford, J. & Warry, W. (ND). Knowledge transfer/translation project summary report. Available at http://socserv.socsci.mcmaster.ca/ihrktn/ihrkt-images/KTsurveyresults.pdf (accessed November 27, 2009).

Rao, J.K., Alongi, J., Anderson, L.A., Jenkins, L., Stokes, G.-A. & Kane, M. (2005). Development of public health priorities for end-of-life initiatives. *American Journal of Preventive Medicine*, 29(5), 453–460.

Rao, J.K., Anderson, L.A. & Smith, S.M. (2002). End of life is a public health issue. *American Journal of Preventive Medicine*, 23(3), 215–220.

Rogers, W. & Veale, B. (2000). Primary health care and general practice: A scoping report. National Information Service of the General Practice Evaluation Program, Flinders University, South Australia.

Rosenberg, J. (1992). Palliative care in the home—a surprising component of Primary Health Care? Paper presented at the Primary Health Care: Development and Diversity Conference, Sydney.

Rosenberg, J.P. (2007). A study of the integration of health promotion principles and practice in palliative care organisations. Queensland University of Technology, Brisbane.

Rosenberg, J.P. & Yates, P.M. (2010a). Health promotion and palliative care: The case for conceptual congruence. *Critical Public Health*, (in press).

Rosenberg, J.P. & Yates, P.M. (2010b). Transition from conventional to health promoting palliative care: An Australian case study. In: Conway, S. (ed.) *Governing Death and Loss: Empowerment, Involvement and Participation* (in press).

Wakerman, J. (2009). Innovative rural and remote primary health care models: What do we know and what are the research priorities? *Australian Journal of Rural Health*, 17(1): 21–26.

Wass, A. (2000). *Promoting Health*. Marrickville, NSW: Elsevier.

World Health Organization (WHO) (1978). Declaration of Alma-Ata. International Conference on Primary Health Care, Alma-Ata, USSR, 6–12 September 1978. Available at http://www.who.int/hpr/NPH/docs/declaration_almaata.pdf (accessed November 27, 2009).

World Health Organization (WHO) (2007). *People at the Centre of Health Care: Harmonizing Mind and Body, People and Systems*. Geneva: WHO Regional Office for South-East Asia and WHO Regional Office for the Western Pacific.

Chapter 4

Making context work in acute care

Alison Hutchinson and Tracey Bucknall

Introduction

The importance of the context of practice to the quality of care delivered has been established in prior chapters and is no less important in the acute care setting. The term "acute care" generally refers to care delivered within a hospital (Mosby's Medical Dictionary, 2009). For the purposes of this chapter, "acute care" includes secondary care, that is, care delivered in hospitals in which routine medical and surgical services are provided, and tertiary care, that is, care delivered in hospitals in which highly specialized and technically advanced services are offered (Green & Bowie, 2005; Lui & Mills, 2007). Typically, tertiary centers are located in major cities while secondary level hospitals may be located in urban or rural areas (Lui & Mills, 2007).

In many countries, hospital services are categorized, according to ownership, into either public or private systems. Public sector hospitals are the responsibility of federal and/or state or provincial governments and are funded by taxpayer dollars. Private sector hospitals, on the other hand, are predominantly owned by private entities (Lui & Mills, 2007). A further distinction between hospitals, on the basis of financial goals, is applied in some countries. For-profit hospitals generate income for the owners of the organization, while profits generated by not-for-profit hospitals are reinvested in the organization in order to improve facilities or services, for example (Lui & Mills, 2007). Public hospitals fit the not-for-profit category, while private hospitals may be operated as either for-profit or not-for-profit organizations (Lui & Mills, 2007). The system or combination of systems adopted, and the size and numbers of secondary and tertiary hospitals that exist, tend to vary by country (Lui & Mills, 2007).

The purpose of this chapter is to examine the influence of the acute care context on the use of evidence in practice. First, a discussion of the significance of using evidence in the acute care context is presented. This will be followed by an examination of the variety of acute care contexts in which nurses work, and the issues unique to such contexts that confront nurses. The discussion will then turn to an examination of empirical evidence on the influence of the acute care context on nurses' use of research evidence in practice. Following this we will discuss types of interventions and important considerations for strategies to promote evidence-based practice. Finally, an example of an implementation strategy used to facilitate the uptake of an evidence-based guideline will be presented.

The acute care context in relation to use of evidence in practice

The importance of using evidence to inform practice has been discussed throughout the nursing literature for over three decades. The reason for repeated reference to, and escalating concern about, this issue is the failure of health professionals, including nurses, to integrate scientific research findings into their practice in a timely manner. This phenomenon is frequently referred to as the research–practice gap or, as Estabrooks describes it, the "gap that exists between what nurses know (research) and what nurses do (practice)" (Estabrooks, 1999b, p. 203). The significance of the delay in integrating research evidence into practice relates to the lost opportunity for the recipients of health care to benefit from the best available evidence, and the consequences, for them and the community, of the delivery of suboptimal care. The underlying assumption, of course, is that delivery of care based upon the best available evidence will result in superior health outcomes for patients. The body of empirical evidence demonstrating improved health care outcomes in response to the delivery of research-based practice continues to expand (Balogh et al., 2005; Barr et al., 2004; Beaupre et al., 2006; Heater et al., 1988).

Early research undertaken to identify reasons for the existence of the research–practice gap focused on characteristics of the individual (Champion & Leach, 1989; Coyle & Sokop, 1990;

Estabrooks et al., 2003; Michel & Sneed, 1995; Rodgers, 2000). More recently, the context in which health professionals practice has received increasing attention from researchers studying the uptake of research evidence. Estabrooks (1999b) describes the organizational determinants of research utilization as "those characteristics of health-care organizations, or units within those institutions, and of governance structures outside of those institutions that facilitate the dissemination and uptake of research findings" (Estabrooks, 1999a, p. 61). More recently, Estabrooks and colleagues (2008) have argued that the lack of positive findings from studies examining interventions to increase research uptake is the result of failure to consider the influence of contextual factors on research use.

In developing a framework to promote the implementation of research in health services, the importance of the context of practice was acknowledged as an essential element (Kitson et al., 1998; Rycroft-Malone, 2004). Defined as "the environment or setting in which the proposed change is to be implemented" (Kitson et al., 1998, p. 150), context is conceived by the investigators as comprising the dimensions of culture, leadership, and evaluation. In a subsequent concept analysis, as outlined in Chapter 2, the researchers define culture as a continuum based on the degree of clarity in values and beliefs, the level of regard for individuals, the organizational drive (task versus learning), the degree of consistency in valuing relationships, teamwork, power, and authority, and the extent of recognition or reward that is provided (McCormack et al., 2002). The leadership continuum is a function of leadership style, role clarity, level of teamwork, effectiveness of organizational structures, decision-making processes, and approaches to teaching, learning, and management (McCormack et al., 2002). Evaluation is also conceived to exist on a continuum, which is determined by the extent of performance feedback provided, the sources of information used to measure performance, and the number of methods used in the process of evaluation (McCormack et al., 2002). The researchers note that the settings, communities and cultures in which health care is delivered are subject to the influences of a range of factors including, but not limited to, economic forces, social influences, political forces, and historical patterns. Hence, the possible range of contexts arising from varying combinations and levels of such influences is inconceivable (McCormack et al., 2002).

Characteristics of acute care contexts

There is a range of structural, procedural, and interprofessional factors that vary in accordance with the context of acute care delivery and have the potential to affect the ease and success of research uptake. In developed countries, acute care hospitals are traditionally comprised of separate specialty-specific wards. Such wards are frequently classified and configured according to a systems approach to health care and include specialties such as neuroscience, nephrology, coronary care, urology, orthopedics, gastroenterology, and the list goes on. Other wards and units may be classified according to disease types, for example, oncology units that specialize in the care of patients diagnosed with cancers. Additionally, highly specialized units, such as critical or intensive care, cardiothoracic surgery, emergency care and perioperative care units, exist to provide highly technical and specialized care to specific groups of patients. Regardless of the practice area, the acute care setting tends to be characterized by complexity, a high rate of change, and unpredictability.

Patients are admitted to acute care hospitals either electively or in need of emergency treatment. Different wards, dependent on their specialty, tend to receive differing mixes of elective and emergency admissions. Often wards are designated to predominantly receive elective patients, such as day of surgery patients, while other wards are designated to receive patients from the emergency department. In the busy hospital setting, there is usually an expectation, however, that flexibility regarding admission practices be exercised, thereby enabling a patient who would ideally be admitted to a specific ward, in the event that a bed is not available, to be admitted to an alternative ward. Such circumstances can create additional pressures for nursing staff who are required to care for patients with conditions for which they have limited knowledge or experience (Duffield et al., 2007). Additionally, the nurses in this situation are required to liaise with medical and allied health professionals who are often unfamiliar and frequently less accessible than are the medical and allied health professionals closely affiliated with their ward or unit.

The organization of care delivery employed within a ward or unit may differ according to the setting. For example, in an intensive care unit a nurse will generally be responsible for the care of one or two patients, while in a general ward the nurse may be responsible for the care of several patients at any one time. In some countries registered nurses may also supervise the delivery of direct patient care by nurses who have received a lower level of education. Dependent on the jurisdiction, these nurses are referred to as licensed practical nurses, licensed vocational nurses, enrolled nurses, and Division 2 nurses, amongst other titles. Different models or approaches to the organization and delivery of care may be adopted. For example, a team approach may be employed, whereby two or more nurses work together to deliver care to a defined number of patients. Alternatively, a primary nursing care model may be used, according to which a nurse assumes the role of primary nurse for individual patients and in doing so accepts responsibility and authority for the coordination of the care for those patients for the duration of their admission (Manthey, 2009), with the goal of maximizing continuity of care.

In the delivery of patient care, nurses interact with a variety of other health professionals and ancillary staff to varying degrees, dependent upon the setting. For instance, in the intensive care setting, nurses work closely with physicians and respiratory therapists and/or physiotherapists in the delivery of patient care. In the oncology setting, nurses are likely to work closely with physicians, dieticians, social workers, and physiotherapists. Additionally, nurses interact with catering, cleaning, administrative, and other support service staff. Thus, in the delivery of care, nurses do not function independently of other professional groups and categories of staff, and therefore the process of nursing care delivery is necessarily influenced, and often complicated or even restricted, by the practices, routines, and processes employed by other health professionals and categories of staff.

Evidence of the influence of acute care context on the use of research in practice

To date, few studies have examined the influence of the acute care context on nurses' use of research in their practice. In an early study that involved the implementation of evidence-based changes in mouth care and preoperative fasting practices in acute care settings, Hunt (1987) found that uptake of these practices occurred to different degrees across units. This study illustrates some of the characteristics of the context of practice that need to be addressed and some of the barriers that need to be overcome in order to successfully implement change in the acute care setting.

Leadership was one aspect of context that influenced the extent to which the evidence was adopted in different units (Hunt, 1987). Namely, not all unit (ward) managers complied with the newly disseminated guidelines on mouth care and, therefore, differential uptake of the practice occurred across units. Additionally, the interrelationship between a range of settings and disciplines, and the coordination and cooperation between them that was required to effect change, presented a challenging and complex barrier to change (Hunt, 1987). Specifically, in order to introduce evidence-based preoperative fasting practices, consultation with surgeons was necessary to formulate and achieve consensus on the guidelines. The guidelines then had to be formally evaluated and authorized by the Procedure Committee, following which they were disseminated to the unit managers. However, implementation at the unit level was complicated, initially, by unpredictable surgery schedules. To overcome this, representatives of a range of staff, including operating room staff, ward-based staff (including day and night staff), surgeons, catering, and housekeeping staff had to work cooperatively to establish a strategy to integrate the change into practice. The impact of this change on nurses' work routines meant that nurses had the greatest difficulties in adopting the change. These difficulties were further compounded by the physical layouts of the wards, which did not readily lend themselves to a change in food and beverage delivery and collection routines (Hunt, 1987). This early work by Hunt provides evidence of the importance of context in successfully integrating evidence into practice.

In 2006, Meijers and colleagues undertook a systematic review to assess the relationships between characteristics of context and research utilization. They found six contextual factors to have a statistically significant relationship with research use, including (1) the role of the nurse, (2) multifaceted access to resources (human, material, and research-related), (3) the organizational climate, (4) multifaceted support (human support, material support, and support for the conduct of research), (5) time for research activities, and (6) the provision of education. The researchers concluded that because "the environments within which nurses work are so complex, multi-faceted and varied" (p. 632), measurement of the context of nursing work is challenging.

In a study of nurses working in the acute care setting in Alberta, Canada, Cummings and colleagues (2007) found organizational characteristics that were positively associated with research utilization included staff development, opportunity for nurse-to-nurse collaboration, and staffing and support services. Furthermore, nurses working in settings in which perceptions of culture, leadership, and evaluation (variables used to measure the PARiHS dimensions of context, outlined in Chapter 2) were more positive, and also reported higher levels of research use and staff development when compared with their colleagues who had less positive perceptions of the contexts in which they worked.

More recently, an exploratory study undertaken by Estabrooks and colleagues (2008) examined the influence of unit-level acute care contextual factors on nurses' use of research in practice. The researchers' intent was to identify the contextual determinants of research use in acute care hospitals. Further, they aimed to model the quintessential acute care unit, possessing the features required to maximize the use of best available evidence. Based on nurses' self-reported data, aggregated to the unit level, the units with the highest levels of research use were also associated with the highest mean scores for self-reported critical thinking dispositions and the highest mean scores for unit culture. In this study, unit culture was evaluated according to five subscales comprising support from co-workers, questioning behavior, access to continuing education, work values related to creativity, and work values related to efficiency. Such characteristics are potentially amenable to change and, therefore, could be modified to increase the use of research in the delivery of health care. Estabrooks and colleagues' findings provide empirical evidence for the influence of contextual factors, in the acute care setting, on the adoption of research in practice.

Interventions and strategies to implement interventions

In this section interventions to promote the use of evidence in practice and strategies to maximize the success of such interventions will be discussed. The success of an intervention is contingent upon a systematically planned and meticulously executed implementation strategy. However, the strategy must allow for flexibility, particularly in environments that are highly demanding and subject to frequent and often unexpected change. A further important consideration for any intervention is whether it will be sustainable. An intervention that is unrealistically costly, or demands resources that are prohibitively expensive, or are inaccessible, is not sustainable and, therefore, should not be implemented. It is imperative that sustainability of the intervention is carefully thought through and, if necessary, that modifications are made to ensure that it is realistic and offers a long-term solution.

For the purposes of this discussion, interventions include the specific components or mechanisms used to integrate evidence into practice, while strategies comprise the support structure and processes that are put in place to help effect the intervention-induced change. Evidence may be incorporated into clinical management tools such as clinical practice guidelines, policies, procedures, and clinical pathways. Interventions may then be put in place to promote the adoption of the respective tools. For examples of interventions employed to integrate evidence into practice, see Box 4.1. Interventions may be delivered at various levels including the micro or individual level, at the meso- or organizational level, and at the macro- or wider societal level. Within an implementation strategy, multiple interventions may be included to target one or more levels.

Systematic reviews examining the evidence for the effectiveness of such interventions in health care, including audit and feedback, reminders, and outreach visiting, have found that they are effective to varying degrees in some, but not all circumstances. Given the

---

Box 4.1 Interventions used to integrate evidence into practice

Local consensus projects

Audit and feedback

Education—distribution of educational material, conferences, self-learning packages

Reminders

Opinion leaders

Educational outreach

External facilitator

Academic detailing

Patient-mediated interventions—e.g., information material

Peer review

Incentives/rewards

Storytelling

inconsistent findings regarding the effectiveness of such interventions, it is difficult to determine the circumstances under which they are likely to be effective (The Improved Clinical Effectiveness through Behavioural Research Group, 2006). Thompson and colleagues (2007) published a systematic review of interventions aimed at increasing use of research in nursing. The most commonly reported intervention they found was education. Educational meetings that were led by a researcher were ineffective in two studies. However, educational meetings led by a local opinion leader and the formation of a multidisciplinary committee were effective in terms of increasing research use in one study each. Thompson and colleagues concluded that little is currently known about how to increase the use of research in nursing and "the evidence to support or refute specific interventions is inconclusive" (Abstract, Conclusion). According to Thompson and colleagues, educational meetings "of varying content, duration and frequency cannot be said to be effective research utilization interventions in nursing" (Findings, paragraph 5). The researchers recommended more rigorous examination or investigation of education as an intervention and concluded that the evidence was inconclusive. The complexity of the interventions, and the variation across studies in how the interventions are delivered and measured, have also added to the uncertainty about circumstances in which certain interventions may be effective. Theoretically informed intervention selection and strategy development is one means by which this problem can be overcome, and an understanding of the circumstances most likely to be associated with successful implementation may be achieved (Rycroft-Malone & Bucknall, 2010; The Improved Clinical Effectiveness through Behavioural Research Group, 2006).

Ingredients of successful implementation

Theory-informed interventions

The importance of using theory to inform selection of interventions, strategy formulation, and evaluation mechanisms has been increasingly emphasized in the knowledge translation literature (Eccles et al., 2005; Rycroft-Malone & Bucknall, 2010; Sales et al., 2006; The Improved Clinical Effectiveness through Behavioural Research Group, 2006). Sales and colleagues argue that the use of theory may help in explaining why an intervention is successful. Behaviour change theory, they explain, deals with why individuals or organizations behave in a certain way and, based on this, addresses factors that would stimulate behavior change. Theory selection should be guided by the level at which the behavior change is targeted. So, for example, if individual behavior change is required, behavior change theory may be most appropriate. If, however change is required at the organizational level, communication theory or social marketing theory may be more appropriate. A combination of theories may also be employed, particularly when change at varying levels is required.

Sales and colleagues (2006) acknowledge that practitioners concerned with improving the quality of care may not recognize or appreciate the benefits of using theory, particularly in circumstances that require immediate action. However, failure to use a theoretical framework risks not having insight into how an intervention works, which may result in failure to consider and account for important elements of an intervention and, consequently, may jeopardize the success of the intervention. Sales and colleagues stress that the use of theory is particularly important when targeting individuals who function within complex organizations such as hospitals. Further, they argue for the importance of considering the interaction between the individual and the organization when planning interventions. This is particularly relevant to the acute care context in which multiple staff from a range of categories and disciplines interact across multiple levels within the organization.

In selecting a theory-linked strategy, consideration should be given to the relationship between characteristics that are considered important in theory. For example, *Social Influence Theory*, emerging predominantly from the field of social psychology, facilitates an understanding of how the behavior of one individual influences that of another (Zimbardo & Leippe, 1991). If such a theory were employed in the acute care setting, the implementation strategy may involve the inclusion of regular formal and informal meetings between health professionals with varying disciplinary backgrounds to enable sharing of knowledge and to promote discussion about how they could work together to ensure a particular practice is introduced and maintained. Additionally, an opinion leader might be included in the intervention.

Measurement of practice prior to implementation of an intervention

While anecdotal evidence of current practice often exists, it is crucial that practice-related baseline data measuring and/or describing practitioners' behavior and/or patient outcomes be undertaken prior to implementation of an intervention. This phase is important in that it not only provides objective evidence of the state of current practice, but such evidence can also be used in the process of increasing practitioners' awareness of deficiencies in practice and persuading them of the importance of adopting practice change. Further, such evidence is vital to an evaluation of the success of the intervention in promoting changes in practitioners' behavior and/or patient outcomes. These changes cannot be measured in the absence of baseline data. Unfortunately, however, in the haste to implement change in a busy acute care setting this stage of an implementation strategy is often overlooked, and once the implementation phase has commenced it is very difficult, and often impossible, to collect such information retrospectively.

It is often necessary to purposively design instruments to collect baseline data associated with an issue in practice. Careful and thoughtful attention to developing the instrument will ensure that useful information is collected. An audit tool for chart review, observation of practitioners in practice, and interviews of practitioners and managers are methods that can be considered for collection of baseline data. Consideration should be given to how the information will be analyzed and reported so that superfluous data are not collected. Additionally, the amount of time that will be required to collect the data and who will be undertaking data collection will also need to be determined. These are important issues because collection of baseline data can be a time-consuming process and resources to enable it to occur need to be factored into the overall implementation strategy.

Diagnostic assessment of context

Critical to the success of an intervention to promote evidence-based practice is an intimate understanding of the context into which the evidence is to be integrated. Therefore, to maximize the success of an intervention it is imperative that a diagnostic evaluation be undertaken prior to, or incorporated within, the implementation strategy. The findings of this evaluation can then be used to inform the selection of the intervention/s (Sales et al., 2006). This is an important step in the process of integrating evidence into practice because context-specific issues will be revealed, and an understanding of such issues will enable the practitioners to tailor the intervention accordingly and to craft an implementation strategy that is in-keeping with the context. An assessment of context could involve an examination of factors such as those identified by Meijers and colleagues (2006) as having a statistically significant relationship with research use; these were listed earlier in this chapter. An evaluation of potentially modifiable contextual determinants of research use in the acute care setting, for which Estabrooks and colleagues (2008) found empirical support, could also be included in the context assessment.

A diagnostic assessment will enable identification of potential challenges or barriers to implementation that might be encountered. Preventative measures can then be put in place, or contingencies to overcome barriers can be incorporated into the strategy. Additionally, the evaluation will aid in the discovery of potential facilitators that can be capitalized upon, or even potentiated, to promote the success of the implementation strategy. In examining factors influencing the implementation of best practice guidelines, Ploeg and colleagues (2007) found a range of barriers and facilitators acting at the individual, organizational, and environmental levels and concluded that implementation strategies should take into consideration such influences and be tailored according to the needs of different stakeholders.

The receptiveness or readiness of the context to change can also be assessed during a diagnostic evaluation, and an awareness of this is important because it will inform the design of the implementation strategy. For example, in contexts where practitioners exhibit signs of reticence or openly negative attitudes toward the proposed change, the implementation strategy will need to incorporate more energy and time to provide compelling evidence of the need for, and benefits of, the change. However, if implementing evidence-based change in contexts where practitioners are already convinced of the benefits of the change, less time will need to be spent in convincing practitioners of the need for the change.

The findings of the diagnostic evaluation should inform selection of appropriate intervention/s. The intervention needs to be carefully tailored according to the context in which it is being applied and consideration given to the potential challenges and opportunities identified during the diagnostic assessment. An education intervention, for example, will be highly specific to the content being delivered, the recipients of the education, and the acute care setting to which it pertains.

Based on the selected interventions, context-specific tools will be required. For example, for an audit and feedback intervention to improve pain assessment and management practices by nurses, an audit tool to evaluate pain assessment and management would be tailored according to the specific context in which it is to be used. Audit tools to collect data on *acute* pain assessment and management are likely to differ from those designed to collect data on *chronic* pain assessment and management. Likewise, an audit tool to assess such practices in the pediatric setting will be different to a tool for use in an adult oncology setting because of the nature of the pain assessment instruments and management practices employed in the respective settings. Similarly, to ensure feedback reports are relevant and understandable they should be carefully tailored according to the setting in which they are to be disseminated and the audience to whom they are directed.

Establishment and communication of clear expectations

Practitioners need to have an understanding of the expectations of them and the performance benchmarks and measures that will be used to assess adherence to the intervention. Communication of this information can be undertaken in a number of ways—through presentations, print materials, web-based materials including links to "frequently asked questions," and one-on-one communication, depending on the scale and form of the intervention. In addition, the benchmarks used to measure performance should be clinically meaningful and locally acceptable, or there is a risk that practitioners will consider feedback irrelevant and meaningless (Hagedorn et al., 2006).

Evaluation of the intervention strategy

Evaluation of the success of an intervention strategy is tightly connected to the collection of relevant baseline information, as previously discussed. The collection of evaluation data may involve methods such as chart audit, observation, and interviews with practitioners and other staff affected by the change. Feedback about the ease of using the intervention should also be sought so that any obstacles or frustrations identified by staff can be addressed. The evaluation, generally, should not involve a one-off assessment but should constitute an ongoing process to evaluate, over time, the success of the intervention (Hagedorn et al., 2006). Ongoing, formative, evaluation will identify elements of the practice change to which practitioners are not adhering as well as those to which they are adhering. This information can be used to inform adjustments or enhancements to the implementation strategy to help promote adherence, and also to encourage and congratulate staff regarding the aspects of their practice that have changed in accordance with the intervention.

Application of research evidence in the acute care context—a case example

In the following section we present, by way of an example, an implementation strategy employed in a large, metropolitan, teaching hospital in Australia (Bucknall, 2007). Between 5% and 20% of drug administrations in Australian hospitals result in an error (Australian Council for Safety and Quality in Health Care, 2002). Prompted by these error rates, the Australian Council for Safety and Quality in Health Care (ACSQHC) developed a National Inpatient Medication Chart (NIMC) to provide a common medication documentation system across acute care settings in order to improve communication and the documentation practices of nurses and doctors, with the ultimate aim of reducing medication administration errors. The Australian Health Ministers endorsed the chart and mandated its introduction into all public hospitals (Australian Health Ministers' Conference, 2004).

The purpose of the implementation strategy was to facilitate the acceptance and adoption of the NIMC by practitioners working within the organization concerned. As previously discussed, the acute care setting is characterized by a high degree of complexity, unpredictability, and frequent (and often rapid) change. Further, the organizational context is subject to influences from a range of levels—macro, meso, and micro. In the case of the NIMC, macro-level influences were exerted by the government mandate for implementation and reporting. Further, the Australian Health Ministers set a deadline for implementation by all public hospitals. At the meso-level, senior hospital administrators, in consultation with middle managers, formulated the implementation strategy in accordance with the timelines set by government. Finally, the influences exerted by the macro- and meso-levels aimed to change practice at the micro-level, the individual practitioner.

Complexity science provides a framework for understanding practice change and offers the potential to examine how systems behave in reality, rather than how they ought to behave (Miller et al., 1998).

To this end, we drew on complexity science to help understand the particular evidence-based practice change within the highly varied and complex context in which it was occurring, and to frame the respective implementation and evaluation strategy. According to complexity science, the relationship between the constituent parts of a system are more important than the individual components themselves, and minimum specification, rather than detailed and complicated plans, is more likely to generate creative and innovative ideas and mechanisms to realize the desired change (Plsek & Wilson, 2001). Thus, collaboration between various stakeholders within the organization, rather than targeting parts of the system, is more likely to be successful. Complexity thinking recommends the use of multiple strategies at the outset. Over time, identification of the strategies that prove most successful in the circumstances and context concerned enables the implementation team to concentrate on the use and enhancement of those particular strategies (Zimmerman et al., 1998). Recognizing that the context of practice undergoes constant change and that behavior is unpredictable, complexity science highlights the importance of flexibility and strong leadership to enable adaptation and to constructively deal with resistance to change (Plsek & Wilson, 2001).

A number of strategic initiatives were adopted to effect the change and the multifaceted strategy involved a multistage, iterative process. As a first step a steering group was convened and a project officer was seconded for the project. Four multidisciplinary working groups comprising key stakeholders were established; each led by a member of the steering group. The groups, including the communication, supply, education, and evaluation group, were formed to address four separate but complementary elements of the strategy.

A communication strategy aimed to target all stakeholders across the range of disciplines was formulated. The communication group established processes for the dissemination of information with the goal of ensuring all relevant staff were familiar with the guidelines and understood the documentation requirements. The strategy involved mass and individual communication mechanisms, tailored according to the stage of adoption and the different disciplines involved. Written information was provided in the form of a weekly newsletter and verbal communication occurred at departmental meetings. Audit data collected by the evaluation group were incorporated in the information that was disseminated. The communication strategy included a range of information dissemination mechanisms—e-mail reminders were sent out to staff, decision prompts were provided on the wards, a telephone hotline was established to address questions or concerns, posters to raise awareness were posted in the wards, and a hospital intranet web site, which included answers to "frequently asked questions," was established.

In recognition of the unique requirements of certain institutions, organizations were permitted to add some features to the NIMC template. To this end, the supply group consulted with key stakeholders during interdisciplinary forums to ascertain specific documentation requirements. Such requirements were then crafted in accordance with government requirements. This was an important but lengthy process resulting in a number of iterations of the document as a result of extensive consultation. The supply group was responsible for organizing the printing and supply of the finalized chart and the removal of the obsolete charts from all areas of the organization. The removal of obsolete charts and the distribution of the new charts were conducted en *masse* in one day to ensure that obsolete charts could not be used from that point onward.

The education group formulated and executed an education strategy tailored according to stages of the implementation process and the needs of the different disciplinary groups. This strategy comprised a range of educational approaches including lectures, workshops, and individualized teaching. The education sessions provided staff with information about the significance of medication error rates and the rationale for the introduction of a common chart and guidelines across all hospitals. The audit data collected by the evaluation group were used to inform the education strategy. As such, aspects of documentation in which deficits were identified were specifically targeted during education sessions. PowerPoint presentations were used to visually display information about the documentation requirements and audit data results. The project officer and a team of nurse educators delivered all education sessions. Attendance at an education session was mandatory for all clinical staff.

Using audits, the NIMC documentation practices of medical and nursing staff were evaluated for adoption of, and adherence to, the medication documentation guidelines. A pharmacist and a registered nurse conducted the audits simultaneously, each examining different elements of every audited chart. To establish baseline data, in order to inform the education component of the strategy and to enable ongoing evaluation, a pre-implementation audit of a random selection of inpatient charts from each ward throughout the hospital was undertaken on a single day, 3 months prior to introduction of the chart. Follow-up audit data were collected at 3 and 12 months following introduction of the NIMC. These audit data served to inform ongoing education and feedback sessions, and to measure the extent of adoption of the chart.

Outcomes measured to assess the level of adherence to the required NIMC documentation practices included adherence to the NIMC best practice documentation requirements for prescribing and administration of medications (intermediate outcome), and the hospital medication error rates and causes as reported through the adverse event reporting system (distal outcome). Individual and focus group interviews were conducted with key stakeholders to elicit opinions regarding the implementation process. Consultation with health professionals, to elicit and respond to their concerns about the change, occurred during regular information forums held throughout the implementation process. Communication between professional groups regarding discipline-specific NIMC documentation responsibilities was identified as an area requiring improvement. Strong leadership was identified as highly beneficial in providing strategies and mechanisms for dealing with poor adherence to the documentation requirements. There was also a need for ongoing governance, management, and monitoring.

The results of the project have been used to inform the development of education programs for the orientation of new clinical staff. These results have also informed ongoing education programs for all health professionals to improve medication prescribing and administration practices, and increase awareness of medication errors and their causes. It was hoped that this would promote a culture of professional accountability and questioning of practice in order to minimize medication administration error. Outcomes of the implementation strategy have also been presented at national and international levels to disseminate knowledge acquired and lessons learnt from the implementation process. Questions relating to medication administration using the NIMC have been incorporated into the electronic medication administration competency requirements for nurses. The audit results have also enabled reporting to government on the degree of success of the implementation strategy.

Conclusion

This chapter has examined the influence of the acute care context on the use of evidence in practice. Specifically, we have considered the significance of using evidence in the acute care context, the variety of acute care settings in which nurses work, and the issues particular to such settings that affect nurses' endeavors to ensure an evidential basis for their practice. We have also discussed relevant scientific literature that examines the influence of the acute care context on nurses' use of research evidence in practice. The range of interventions available, and important elements to consider when designing strategies to promote evidence-based practice, has also been explored. The complex and highly demanding nature of the acute care context, which is characterized by unpredictability and constant change, makes attempts to enhance the use of evidence in practice extremely challenging. Nonetheless, the challenge is not insurmountable. Thoughtful planning and communication, coupled with provision for flexibility and adaptability in accordance with a changing health care context, are vital to the success of a strategy to implement evidence into practice in the acute care setting.

References

Australian Council for Safety and Quality in Health Care (2002). Second National Report on Medication Safety. Canberra, Australia: Commonwealth Department of Health.

Australian Health Ministers' Conference (2004). Joint communique. Online. Available at http://www.safetyandquality.gov.au/internet/safety/publishing.nsf/content/F3D3F3274D393DFCCA257483000D8461/$File/chcommun.pdf (accessed June 12, 2009).

Balogh, Z., Caldwell, E., Heetveld, M. et al. (2005). Institutional practice guidelines on management of pelvic fracture-related hemodynamic instability: Do they make a difference? *Journal of Trauma*, 58, 778–782.

Barr, J., Hecht, M., Flavin, K.E., Khorana, A. & Gould, M.K. (2004). Outcomes in critically ill patients before and after the implementation of an evidence-based nutritional management protocol. *Chest*, 125, 1446–1457.

Beaupre, L.A., Cinats, J.G., Senthilselvan, A. et al. (2006). Reduced morbidity for elderly patients with a hip fracture after implementation of a perioperative evidence-based clinical pathway. *Quality and Safety in Health Care*, 15, 375–379.

Bucknall, T.K. (2007). Implementing guidelines to improve medication safety for hospitalised patients: Experiences from Western Health, Australia. *Worldviews on Evidence-Based Nursing*, 4, 51–53.

Champion, V.L. & Leach, A. (1989). Variables related to research utilization in nursing: An empirical investigation. *Journal of Advanced Nursing*, 14, 705–710.

Coyle, L.A. & Sokop, A.G. (1990). Innovation adoption behavior among nurses. *Nursing Research*, 39, 176–180.

Cummings, G.G., Estabrooks, C.A., Midodzi, W.K., Wallin, L. & Hayduk, L. (2007). Influence of organizational characteristics and context on research utilization. *Nursing Research*, 56, S24–S39.

Duffield, C., Roche, M., O'Brien-Pallas. et al. (2007). Glueing it together: Nurses, their work environment and patient safety. Sydney, Australia: University of Technology.

Eccles, M., Grimshaw, J., Walker, A., Johnston, M. & Pitts, N. (2005). Changing the behavior of healthcare professionals: The use of theory in promoting the uptake of research findings. *Journal of Clinical Epidemiology*, 58, 107–112.

Estabrooks, C.A. (1999a). Mapping the research utilization field in nursing. *Canadian Journal of Nursing Research*, 31, 53–72.

Estabrooks, C.A. (1999b). The conceptual structure of research utilization. *Research in Health and Nursing*, 22, 203–216.

Estabrooks, C.A., Floyd, J.A., Scott-Findlay, S., O'Leary, K.A. & Gushta, M. (2003). Individual determinants of research utilization: A systematic review. *Journal of Advanced Nursing*, 43, 506–520.

Estabrooks, C.A., Scott, S., Squires, J.E. et al. (2008). Patterns of research utilization on patient care units. *Implementation Science*, 3, 31. Online. Available at http://www.implementationscience.com/content/3/1/31 (accessed May 17, 2009).

Green, M.A. & Bowie, M.J. (2005). Essentials of health information management. Principles and practices. Clifton Park, NY: CENGAGE Delmar Learning.

Hagedorn, H., Hogan, M., Smith, J.L. et al. (2006). Lessons learned about implementing research evidence into clinical practice experiences from VA QUERI. *Journal of General Internal Medicine*, 21, S21–S24.

Heater, B.S., Becker, A.M. & Olson, R.K. (1988). Nursing interventions and patient outcomes: A meta-analysis of studies. *Nursing Research*, 37, 303–307.

Hunt, M. (1987). The process of translating research findings into nursing practice. *Journal of Advanced Nursing*, 12, 101–110.

Kitson, A., Harvey, G. & McCormack, B. (1998). Enabling the implementation of evidence based practice: A conceptual framework. *Quality in Health Care*, 7, 149–158.

Lui, X. & Mills, A. (2007). Economic models of hospital behavior Washington, DC. In: Preker, A.S., Liu, X., Velenyi, E.V. & Baris, E. (eds) *Public Ends, Private Means. Strategic Purchasing of Health Services*. Washington, DC: The World Bank, pp. 209–236.

Manthey, M. (2009). The 40th anniversary of primary nursing. Setting the record straight. *Creative Nursing*, 15, 36–38.

McCormack, B., Kitson, A., Harvey, G., Rycroft-Malone, J., Titchen, A. & Seers, K. (2002). Getting evidence into practice: The meaning of "context." *Journal of Advanced Nursing*, 38, 94–104.

Meijers, J.M.M., Janssen, M.A.P., Cummings, G.G., Wallin, L., Estabrooks, C.A. & Halfens, R.Y.G. (2006). Assessing the relationships between contextual factors and research utilization in nursing: Systematic literature review. *Journal of Advanced Nursing*, 55, 622–635.

Michel, Y. & Sneed, N.V. (1995). Dissemination and use of research findings in nursing practice. *Journal of Professional Nursing*, 11, 306–311.

Miller, W.L., Crabtree, B.F., McDaniel, R. & Stange, K.C. (1998). Understanding change in primary care practice using complexity theory. *The Journal of Family Practice*, 46, 369–376.

Mosby's Medical Dictionary (2009). 8th ed. Philadelphia, PA: Elsevier.

Ploeg, J., Davies, B., Edwards, N., Gifford, W. & Elliot Miller, P. (2007). Factors influencing best-practice guideline implementation: Lessons learned from administrators, nursing staff, and project leaders. *Worldviews on Evidence-Based Nursing*, 4, 210–219.

Plsek, P.E. & Wilson, T. (2001). Complexity, leadership, and management in healthcare organisations. *British Medical Journal*, 323, 746–749.

Rodgers, S.E. (2000). A study of the utilization of research in practice and the influence of education. *Nurse Education Today*, 20, 273–278.

Rycroft-Malone, J. (2004). The PARIHS framework—a framework for guiding the implementation of evidence-based practice. *Journal of Nursing Care Quality*, 19, 297–304.

Rycroft-Malone, J. and Bucknall, T. (eds.). (2010). Models and Frameworks for Implementing Evidence-Based Practice: Linking Evidence to Action. Oxford, UK: Wiley-Blackwell.

Sales, A., Smith, J., Curran, G. & Kochevar, L. (2006). Models, strategies, and tools. Theory in implementing evidence-based findings into health care practice. *Journal of General Internal Medicine*, 21, S21–S24.

The Improved Clinical Effectiveness through Behavioural Research Group (2006). Designing theoretically-informed implementation interventions. *Implementation Science*, 1, 4. Online. Available at http://www.implementation science.com/content/1/1/4 (accessed May 17, 2009).

Thompson, D.S., Estabrooks, C.A., Scott-Findlay, S., Moore, K. & Wallin, L. (2007). Interventions aimed at increasing research use in nursing: A systematic review. *Implementation Science*, 2, 15. Online. Available at http://www.implementationscience.com/content/2/1/15 (accessed May 17, 2009).

Zimbardo, P.G. & Leippe, M.R. (1991). The psychology of attitude change and social influence. Philadelphia, PA: Temple University Press.

Zimmerman, B.J., Lindberg, C. & Plsek, P.E. (1998). Edgeware: Complexity resources for healthcare leaders. Irving, TX: VHA Publishing.

Chapter 5

Making context work in pediatrics

Valerie Wilson

Introduction

Evidence-based healthcare is an expectation in the 21st century. However, how do we ensure that healthcare environments and healthcare practitioners are best equipped to make sure this is a reality, and that those who receive healthcare and their families are in the best position to advocate for nothing less than this expectation. This chapter will look at evidence-based healthcare within the pediatric context. Whilst many of the issues relating to the delivery of evidence-based healthcare cross the boundaries of contexts and settings such as appraising the evidence, overcoming resistance to change and translating such evidence into practice, there remains some key differences in the pediatric setting which will be touched upon in this chapter.

What sets the pediatric context apart from other contexts such as acute care (Chapter 4) and mental health (Chapter 8) is the type of patient (neonate, child, or young person) receiving healthcare. This includes the developmental and physiological differences within the patient population and the model of care delivery (family centered). There are factors within these two aspects that may be experienced in other healthcare settings, for example, the dependence of the neonate or infant on others for fundamentals such as food, shelter, or personal care may, in a way, be similar to the adult in intensive care or the older person with dementia. It is however the dominance of this as a factor of everyday care within the patient population that stamps it as a context issue for the delivery of pediatric services. We also need to look at the model of family-centered care. While some non-pediatric practitioners would argue that they also deliver family-centered care, by this they often mean that they include the family in discussions about the "patient's care." Family-centered care in pediatrics however is more than this. It encompasses caring for the child in partnership with the family, working with the family to deliver care to the child. What this means in reality, when exploring the contextual factors influencing evidence-based practice in the pediatric setting, will be explored in detail within this chapter.

This chapter will look at these contextual issues using common activities and examples from practice that focus on the uniqueness of the child as well as the model of care delivery and the challenges these aspects hold for those at the heart of practice. There will also be the opportunity to explore the implications of cultural factors that may impact on the delivery of evidence-based pediatric healthcare. The aim is to highlight a number of key considerations for practitioners to think about as part of their own evidence-based practice.

Medication safety

One area of practice that has many implications for the pediatric nurse is that of safe administration of medication to the patient. There is a broad range of evidence that highlights the many factors involved in medication safety. These include systems approaches, such as looking at bar coding and workflow (Koppel et al., 2008), processes such as double checking (Hughes & Edgerton, 2005), to the people involved in administration (doctors, pharmacists, and nurses), and the concept of human error (Reason, 2000) in relation to such things as dosing errors (Kozer, 2009) and "slips in attention" during the prescribing or administration phase (Nichols et al., 2008). Each aspect of this complex activity has been studied and evidence is available to inform us not only about how we go about this frequent activity but also ways in which we can minimize medication-related errors.

A medication error is defined by Hughes and Edgerton (2005) as "preventable, inappropriate use of medications that may occur at any stage of the medication process, including ordering, transcribing orders, dispensing, administering, and monitoring." (p. 79). Expanding on this definition, Wong et al. (2009b) suggest that an error is "any preventable event that may cause or lead to inappropriate medication use or patient harm, while the medication is in the control of the health care professional, patient or consumer. Such events may be related to professional practice, health care products, procedures and systems including: prescribing, order communication, product labelling, packaging and nomenclature, compounding, dispensing, distribution, administration, education, monitoring and use." (p. 161). The similarities between both these definitions is clear, as well as the additional elements introduced in the more recent definition. From these, it is easy to see the potential for error given the complexity of the medication process, the human factor (the different people involved in the process) and the receiver of the medication (the patient).

In the pediatric context, safe medication administration is even more complex given that we are dealing with patients who vary physically (size), physiologically (how drugs are metabolized), in their cognition (their understanding about what the medication is for), and psychologically (their behavior toward medication administration). Children are, therefore, the most vulnerable population and are at greater risk than others because of their immature physiology and physical development (Hughes & Edgerton, 2005), communication challenges (Hughes & Edgerton, 2005; Walsh et al., 2005), and lack of autonomy (Wong et al., 2009a). Those shown to be at most risk are children under 2 years, those who are seriously ill, are in neonatal or pediatric Intensive Care Units (NICU/PICU) or emergency areas (Walsh et al., 2005). Consequently, it is vital that parents are seen as advocates for their children, part of the medication safety process, and feel they are supported and encouraged to ask questions about the medication (Wong et al., 2009a). In addition to this, there is also the necessity of involving parents and preparing them to continue safe administration of medication after discharge. It is therefore of utmost importance to consider the available evidence that helps us to navigate the processes and systems around medication safety and mitigates the potential for error.

Medication errors are the most common adverse event during a child's hospital admission (Hughes & Edgerton, 2005; Wong et al., 2009a) and can lead to significant harm (Wong et al., 2009b). Rates of error are reported to range from 3.9% (Hicks et al., 2007a), as a conservative estimate, to around 5% (Hughes & Edgerton, 2005; Wong et al., 2009b) but may be higher; a study reported that 27% (467) of observed medications administered resulted in an error relating to timing, routes, dosage, unordered drug, or no form (Prot et al., 2005). Errors of course may go unreported (Wong et al.,

2009b), either because they are not detected or there is fear of the consequences of reporting the error (Reason, 2000). Initiatives have been introduced that appear to reduce rates of medication errors; these include bar coding (Koppel et al., 2008) and computerized physician prescribing orders (Kozer, 2009; Taylor et al., 2008; Walsh et al., 2008) although, even with these interventions, medication errors still occurred (Taylor et al., 2008). Fortescue et al. (2003) noted that improvements in communication between doctors and pharmacists and doctors and nurses could have prevented drug errors in the inpatient setting by 47% and 17.4%, respectively. It has also been suggested that most errors occur due to poor attention at any stage in the medication administration process and, most often, these occur after hours, when staff are busy or distracted or when they are unfamiliar with the patient (Nichols et al., 2008).

One area that is of particular importance in the pediatric population relates to dosing errors where the risk is increased due to inaccuracy of the child's weight (Ghaleb & Wong, 2006; Hicks et al., 2007a; Hughes & Edgerton, 2005; McPhillips et al., 2005). This is particularly problematic in neonates, where weights change rapidly and the neonates themselves have limited reserves to cope with any excess of a given drug (Sinha & Cranswick, 2007). Indeed there is debate in the literature about reliance on weight alone in drug calculations; it has been suggested that drug dosage should be based on the child's body surface area (Anderson & Meakin, 2002). Complicating factors relating to dosage errors include miscalculation by staff due to poor maths skills (Hughes & Edgerton, 2005). Misplacement of the decimal point has resulted in 10-fold errors (Hicks et al., 2007a,b; Hughes & Edgerton, 2005; Sinha & Cranswick, 2007; Walsh et al., 2005); these occur more readily in resuscitation situations, given the frenetic nature of the situation (Kozer et al., 2006). Dosing errors, as Sinha and Cranswick (2007) point out, may be compounded by the fact that drugs are often only available in adult packages, and these drugs may need to be diluted (Hughes & Edgerton, 2005; Sinha & Cranswick, 2007), which can lead to errors especially when using inaccurate measuring devices (Sinha & Cranswick, 2007).

It is clear to see, from the evidence, that medication safety in the pediatric context is multifaceted and involves multiple professions. The plethora of evidence we have available regarding this issue is useful in that it provides ample guidance about what we need to pay attention to in order to ensure we have the best chance of delivering medication to children, which is both efficacious and safe.

Table 5.1 Recommendations for safe practice (medications)

- Clear written medications, write down and verify verbal orders (Hughes & Edgerton, 2005)
- Awareness of rules, policies, and guidelines (Hughes & Edgerton, 2005; Sinha & Cranswick, 2007)
- Know about the medication you are going to administer (Hughes & Edgerton, 2005)
- Minimize distractions during all phases of medication administration (Hughes & Edgerton, 2005; Nichols et al., 2008)
- Accurate weight for patient is recorded on chart (Anderson & Meakin, 2002)
- Double check medications (pay careful attention to calculations) (Hughes & Edgerton, 2005; Wong et al., 2009b)
- Be aware that 10-fold errors more likely to occur in resuscitation situations (Kozer et al., 2006)
- Effective communication (amongst staff, patients, and families) (Hughes & Edgerton, 2005; Walsh et al., 2005)
- Confirm patient information before administration (Hughes & Edgerton, 2005; Taylor et al., 2008; Wong et al, 2009b)
- Support parents to advocate for their child (Walsh et al., 2005)
- Open and fair culture where staff feel able to report errors (Hughes & Edgerton, 2005; Reason, 2000; Stephenson, 2005)

Table 5.1 builds on the safety five Rs (right patient, right time and frequency, right dose, right route, right drug) and provides a number of recommendations, sourced from the evidence, that help with reflecting on practice and to think critically about whether practice is evidence based in relation to safe administration of medication to children.

Evidence from practice

The following is a nurse's story (in her own words) taken from clinical practice about medication safety that captures many of the challenges facing nurses everyday in the pediatric setting.

I was working in the nursery that day. When preparing an intramuscular injection of gentamycin with another staff member I discovered that common practice was to dilute the drug to make calculation simpler, as the dose required was very small (that sounded credible). I questioned this practice however as the baby would be receiving a larger volume (× 4) of fluid, and this would make the injection even more painful. I was told that it was the "policy," the drug was toxic and therefore needed to be diluted to reduce toxicity. I knew this "fact" about toxicity was incorrect and, when we looked for the "policy," there was no policy to be found. As I explored the rationale for this practice with the other nurse we realised that this was a long term practice, based on rituals and myth rather than on evidence. We discussed the impact of the injection on the baby, and together we sought further information by ringing other units to find out about their practice (benchmarking); we also sourced information from the pharmacist about the drug and the perceived "toxicity." The outcome was that the drug was not diluted, the baby did receive his medication (albeit thirty minutes later) and practice on the unit was changed, staff no longer followed a fictional policy.

So let us consider some reflective questions arising from this scenario:

- What medication safety risks can be identified?
- What sources of evidence did staff in the nursery use to inform their initial practice?
- What kinds of evidence could be sought to inform or change practice?

There are also some reflective questions that we might want to ask about our practice (Box 5.1):

- What are the guidelines for medication administration in the organization?
- What evidence is used to inform practice around medication safety?

It can be seen from this discussion on medication safety that there are many factors to consider when using evidence to inform practice. The complexity of medication administration results in a myriad of evidence-based decisions and actions that need to be taken by all those involved in the process to ensure that practice is safe. It is, therefore, no surprise that any break in the decision/action process can result in unsafe practice. There is still much work to be done to ensure that evidence is used consistently at each step of the medication administration process (and to inform the systems that support the process) and by each person involved in the process; only then will medication administration be a safer practice.

> **Box 5.1 Interesting facts**
>
> Did you know that some of the drugs we use in the pediatric setting have not been tested for safe use in children (Bonati et al., 1999). Recent studies in Europe have identified that many children admitted to hospital receive drugs that are unlicensed (Conroy et al., 2000); this means that we are not aware of the safety in relation to dose and toxicity and use guesstimates in prescribing (Baber & Pritchard, 2003; Turner et al., 1999).
>
> There is also the additional problem that drugs often come prepared in adult doses and are then required to be reconstituted for the child thereby increasing the risk of calculation and dispensing errors (Chapell & Newman, 2004, Walsh et al., 2005).
>
> In December 2007 the World Health Organization launched a campaign "make medicines child sized" in a bid to raise awareness about this issue and speed up action to resolve it.
>
> They suggest that, to achieve this, more research (evidence) is required.

Overcoming the barriers to implementing evidence into practice

The issues identified when exploring medication safety reveal that there are often barriers that need to be overcome to ensure that evidence is informing or changing practice. We will now explore, using a case example taken from a small action research project "A 'wee' problem" (Smith et al., 2009), some solutions to such barriers.

A systematic review of urine collection mechanisms, commissioned by the National Institute for Health and Clinical Excellence (NICE), recommended that urine pads should be used, in preference to using invasive procedures such as supra-pubic aspirate, if a clean catch specimen is not possible to be obtained (National Collaborating Centre for Women's and Children's Health, 2007). Commonly urine bags are used and although they are classified as "noninvasive" (Ahmad et al., 1991; McKune, 1989), the bags are often found to leak, frequently resulting in excoriation, and require many applications to obtain a sample (McKune, 1989; Waddington & Watson, 1997), which can be distressing for the child (Cohen, 1997). The action research project (A Wee Problem) arose from a sense of frustration around the difficulty of implementing research evidence into practice. The nurse manager in the ward, who took on the role of project leader, had previous experience of using the recommended pads in another setting. She also had an excellent understanding of the research evidence about the use of urine pads, as well as evidence from current practice that highlighted the distress for babies (and parents) when a urine bag was applied or removed to obtain a urine sample. What she had not foreseen, however, were the barriers that had to be overcome in order to get the evidence into and sustained in practice.

The barriers included the following:

- a lack of organizational support
- the pads were more expensive than the bags
- the pads were not easily obtained through a supplier and therefore getting a ready supply was challenging
- challenges in engaging staff in the change process, especially as they were being asked to change from a well-established mechanism for collecting urine samples from babies to a new way of doing things.

There are very strong reasons for translating research evidence into practice in healthcare systems that pursue the notion of best practice and excellence in care delivery (Rycroft-Malone, 2004a). However, there is also an acknowledgment that there are barriers to be overcome (Newman et al., 1998; Retsas, 2000), just as we found when introducing a new way of collecting urine specimens. Whilst there has been a focus on looking at people as barriers (e.g., nurses—McCaughan et al., 2002; Thompson et al., 2001), there is a growing recognition of the complexity of this process and consideration must be made of such things as the culture of the organization, politics, red tape, and social relationships in the workplace (Rycroft-Malone, 2004a). One way of overcoming potential barriers is to include stakeholders, who may be impacted by the change, in the process from the beginning (Harvey et al., 2002). Therefore adopting an approach that is participatory in nature and aimed at facilitating an evidence-based change in practice is vital; for this reason we adopted an action research framework in the urine pad study. The key barriers to overcome were the lack of infrastructure support, lack of stakeholder buy-in, and perceived lack of authority to change practice; all of which have been identified as common barriers in translating evidence into practice (Sams et al., 2004).

With this knowledge in hand, the project team sought wider consultation with a broad range of staff, which highlighted the need to start off small and ensure the change process could be trialled within clinical areas where:

- the team had already established clinical credibility
- urine collection from babies was a common activity
- there was recognition of the problem.

Each of these aspects contributed to a more effective approach to stakeholder engagement. However, it was still recognized that the weight of published evidence alone does not automatically lead to a change in practice. Consequently, active facilitation (to engage stakeholders in the change process) was used since previously it had been suggested as a prerequisite for effective changes in practice (Harvey et al., 2002; Rycroft-Malone et al., 2002). However, for it to be effective, facilitation needs to be combined with understanding the context in which the change is to take place, in this instance two pediatric wards, and the evidence for the change. In Chapter 2, the framework called Promoting Action on Research Implementation in Health Services (PARiHS) was described and it was used here to guide the implementation of evidence-based practice, since it makes explicit the relationship between the type of evidence, the context into which it is being implemented and the facilitation required for change to be successful (Rycroft-Malone, 2004b).

As we experienced in the pad study, effective change can be actively facilitated by working with the relationship between evidence and context, and whilst this is not necessarily easy, it can be achieved. In the following extract, the researchers' reflections on their experience of implementing change and the challenges they faced are captured:

> We naively assumed that what we perceived as a problem to be resolved would automatically be perceived as a problem by others, an assumption which initially inhibited stakeholder consultation in clinical areas where our credibility was less well established. Feeling challenged led us to reflect upon where our circle of influence truly lay and with whom we might most effectively work in order to facilitate a change in practice. This challenge was beneficial to the outcome of the project because it brought about a reflective process that refined our aims, methods and expected outcomes. As uncomfortable as the period of challenge was, it

was crucial to the success of the project. In future we may learn to welcome the discomfort and instability that such challenge brings because it can lead to positive outcomes for the project.

(Smith et al., 2009, p. 18)

Clearly, implementing evidence into practice is neither straightforward nor easy. However, understanding the potential barriers to change and working with the relationship between facilitation, evidence and context will, hopefully, increase the chances of being successful in changing practice. The outcomes from the "wee" project were that nurses in the study sites did identify urine pads as their preferred mechanism for collecting urine, therefore changing their practice, and organizational support was given to ensure a consistent supply of the pads became available. A flow-on effect from this was that nurses in other clinical units adopted the use of pads in their practice—see Smith et al. (2009) for further information.

However, a key reflection arising from the project was the need for a more explicit model of care to be in place in order to ensure greater consistency in practice and the adoption of evidence (such as that in the "wee" project) in care decisions. The final section of this chapter focuses on the model of care delivery in the pediatric setting (family-centered care), and the challenges of ensuring that evidence informs not just what we say we do, but what we actually do in everyday practice.

Family-centered care

The philosophy of care most associated with the pediatric context is family-centered care. If you ask nursing staff in pediatric hospitals, or in pediatric wards in general hospitals, about the care they deliver most of them would be able to tell you about family-centered care. Therefore we can say that the evidence about the importance of family-centered care has definitely been translated into practice in many parts of the world.

The philosophy of family-centered care is not new (Ahmann, 1994; Bradley & Wiggins, 1983; Brown & Ritchie, 1989; Cox, 1974; Darbyshire, 1994; Johnson & Lindschau, 1996; Lee, 2007; O'Connor et al., 1980; Petersen et al., 2004; Ramos, 1992; Shelton et al., 1987; Van Riper, 2001). However, there is confusion arising from the plethora of names given to the principles of care that underpin this approach; these include family-centered care (Shelton et al., 1987); shared care (Keatinge & Gilmore, 1996); parental involvement in care (Hart, 1979); parental partnership in care (Johnson & Lindschau, 1996); the Nottingham model (Smith, 1995); NIDCAP (Als, 1986), and others. This has resulted in uncertainty around the concepts of family-centered care among practitioners and lack of clear guidelines for implementation (Bradley, 1996; Coyne, 1996; Hutchfield, 1999).

Where adopted, family-centered care has been somewhat successful in helping to ensure that parents are now, more than ever, a part of their child's care during hospitalization (Callery & Smith, 1991; Coyne & Cowley, 2007; Daneman et al., 2003; Knight, 1995; Lee, 2007). However, there have been many barriers to successful implementation, including:

- nurses' attitudes (Fisher et al., 2008; Gill, 1987; Johnson & Lindschau, 1996; Lee, 2007; Newton, 2000; Rushton & Glover, 1990; Trnobranski, 1994)
- fear of losing control (Fenwick et al., 2001)
- the technical nature of the environment (Gordin & Johnson, 1999; McGrath, 2000)
- the discrepancy between what we say we do and what we achieve in practice (Fisher et al., 2008; Petersen et al., 2004).

All of these impact upon sustaining changes in practice. Whilst nurses understand and subscribe to the notion of family-centered care, they have found it difficult to embed the principles in practice (Petersen et al., 2004). In other words, they know the evidence and what it says about effective care delivery to children and their families, but they are often unable to translate such evidence into their everyday practice. Therefore, knowing the evidence is not enough in itself to change practice; success is more likely when deep-rooted personal change drives practice innovation (Balfour & Clarke, 2001).

To illustrate this, an example will be used from a research project that focused on realizing a family-centered care model in a special care nursery (SCN) (Wilson, 2005). This work was supported by a facilitator who helped staff understand their practice context, review the evidence base for best practice, examine the ways in which they were working, and how these supported or hindered a family-centered approach to care. These initiatives enabled staff to develop strategies for overcoming some of the barriers to implementation of changes in practice.

Whilst the underpinning philosophy of care delivery in the SCN was said to be based on the principles of family-centered care, there was practice evidence, sourced from observation, staff interviews, and surveys (see Wilson et al., 2005 for further details), of variations in care delivery, disempowering practice and an image of busyness (see Table 5.2). This detracted from the efforts of family-centered practitioners and created a tension between them and staff who favored a nurse-centered approach to care. Whilst nurses in the SCN espoused a philosophy of family-centered care, there was inconsistency in translating this into practice, which resulted in a disorganized approach to care delivery.

In order to illustrate how nursing staff in this context worked through these tensions, used evidence in and about their practice to help them critically look at what was happening, and to inform change, two examples will be used; empowering families and changing the environment of the SCN. Staff in the SCN had access to a variety of activities (action learning, workshops on evidences-based practice, and family-centered care, working with the facilitator in challenging assumptions about practice) to enable them to critically review and reflect on their practice, appraise the evidence–practice gap, and to decide what changes would be required if they were to achieve

Table 5.2 The tensions evident between differing values and beliefs within the culture

Family-centered care		
Empowerment of families	T	*Ownership of babies*
• I see myself as a copartner in the babies care, mums need to feel it's their baby	E	• Focus is on babies in my care . . . look after my babies
Continuity	N	*Discontinuity*
• Continuity of care increases parental confidence	S	• Some involve parents, others find it hard and just want to do it themselves
Enabling environments	I	*Busyness*
• Environments need to be less clinical and optimal for growth	O	• The image of busyness, parents don't want to disturb staff, staff remove cot covers, there are lights 24 h a day, noise levels are high
	N	

family-centered care as an everyday reality. Evidence from the literature has also been used to highlight key points about the existing and changing context of the SCN and the voices of staff (obtained through staff interviews) are embedded within the story in *italics*.

Empowering families

Staff on the SCN had advocated for a model of care that focused on empowering families; however, there was, at that time, evidence of a culture that sent mixed messages to families. The staff's actions influenced family involvement (both positively and negatively), factors that have also been identified in a study by Power and Franck (2008). Behavior and language sometimes served to distance rather than include families (Fenwick et al., 2001; Lightbody, 2009), and nurses were known to take on a paternalistic role (Maxton, 1997; Newton, 2000). Families were also viewed as an adjunct, rather than fundamental to delivery of care, and parental participation was usually based on nurses working on rather than working with parents (Callery & Smith, 1991; Casey, 1995; Daneman, 2003; Knight, 1995; Rushton & Glover, 1990). As had been identified in the literature, some nurses believed that dealing with families interfered with the care of the patient (Bratt et al., 2000; Brown & Ritchie, 1989; Clark & Carter, 2002; Fenwick et al., 2001; Lightbody, 2009; McGrath, 2001). The concept of empowering families should indicate that patients are at the center of care, and yet the evidence arising from the behavior of nurses indicated that they themselves, just as in other studies, were the center of care delivery (Casey, 1995). The findings from the study agreed with those of Caty et al. (2001) who suggested that whilst nurses have good knowledge of family-centered care principles, they are unable to consistently implement them in practice as they have difficulty moving from a "medical helping" model to an "enabling model" which is the foundation of family-centered care.

During the project, staff worked hard to overcome the barriers to empowerment and to shift the focus of care from what was predominantly a nurse-centered model to one that was focused on the family, with the empowerment of parents where *most staff are pretty big on getting the family involved*. This included *involving parents in the decision making* ensuring that care was primarily for the baby *but at the heart of the family unit* and that families were made to *feel it's their baby and it is not ours.* Each of these factors is important in creating a climate that supports collaboration (Eckle & MacLean, 2001; Fenwick et al., 1999; Paavilainen & Astedt-Kurkl, 1997; Rowe & Jones, 2008). There was also an emphasis on including the father in care *it's not just the mother looking after the babies it's also the father* and enabling fathers to become more involved in feeding, bathing, and comforting their baby thereby achieving a level of normality within the care context (Fisher, 2001).

Nurses have been found to be involved in educating parents and openly encouraging them to become involved with their baby in order to facilitate a shared approach to care (Fegran et al., 2008; Johnson & Lindschau, 1996; Keatinge & Gilmore, 1996; Newton, 2000). However, changes that were evident in care in the SCN were not universally adopted and a very small group of nurses persisted in judgmental behavior, which resulted in distancing themselves from the families and focusing their attention on the baby in their care, just as was found in other studies (Bratt et al., 2000; Brown & Ritchie, 1989; Callery & Smith, 1991; Clark & Carter, 2002; Daneman et al., 2003; Fenwick et al., 2001; Knight, 1995; McGrath, 2001). They assumed "the maternal role" (Maxton, 1997). This attitude however was challenged by other staff members and, in the SCN study, their influence on the overall delivery of care was minimal.

Nurses also recognized the multidimensional aspects of family-centered care

> it is also being able to give the emotional support, social support . . . which to me is important . . . it is just as important as delivering care . . . what I like about it is being able to involve the parents, the grandparents . . . involving parents, educating them, embracing them, welcoming them.

These factors have been identified as important to the delivery of family-centered care (Bruce & Ritchie, 1997; Johnson et al., 1992). Welcoming families into the unit has been found to be very important especially during the admission process as first impressions often set the scene for the future care (Newton, 2000). Fenwick et al. (2001) suggest that "language acts as a powerful clinical tool that can be used to assist parents in gaining confidence in caring for their infants and in becoming connected to infants resident in the nursery" (p. 583). Families in the SCN were made to feel comfortable in the environment as nurses considered how they *speak to people* and displayed positive welcoming behaviors such as smiling, introducing themselves, giving parents a chair to sit by the baby, explaining what is going on with the baby, and answering questions. This change in attitudes toward parents meant they were more willing to become actively involved in care, to ask questions, and to be part of the decision-making team (Casey, 1995; Daneman et al., 2003; Eckle & MacLean, 2001; Lee, 2007; Newton, 2000; Rowe & Jones, 2008; Rushton & Glover, 1990; Trnobranski, 1994). Nurses were more aware of how *parents were feeling* about having a sick baby in the SCN environment (Davis et al., 2003; Fisher, 2001) and they realized that *although the baby is the patient, it is the parents you are caring for as well.*

Family-centered environment

Tension existed in the SCN between the *image of busyness* portrayed by some staff members and the desire for an *enabling environment* that supports the growing child and the family (see Table 5.2 for further details). The resulting chaos left parents unsure of their role within the unit and open to the mixed messages conveyed by staff. Care delivery was inconsistent and babies were often subjected to a high level of environmental insult (such as light and noise) and not much in the way of appropriate developmental care. Robinson (2003) suggests that without consistent leadership and clear lines of accountability, developmental care is dependent on the beliefs of the individual, under such circumstances the quality of care is inconsistent and is often unpredictable. The environment of the SCN, unlike the womb, is characterized by loud and unpredictable noise (Lotas, 1992). This is especially problematic for the premature neonate who lacks the mature function to deal with such trauma (Zahr & Balian, 1995). Noise is noxious and has been shown to have detrimental physiological effects on the premature infant (Catlett & Holditch-Davis, 1990) which can result in poor weight gain and reduced healing (Bremmer et al., 2003).

In recent years, staff in the SCN had been striving to improve the environment for the premature and sick neonate in order to improve outcomes (Bowie et al., 2003). These issues were raised by staff and subsequently became one of the major areas of change within the unit. Staff awareness of the evidence related to these issues was highlighted through undertaking literature searches, use of evidence to inform practice changes, challenge and support of one another, staff education, and environmental advocates; all of which are strategies that help facilitate the introduction of developmental care (Perkins et al., 2004). This has resulted in a more developmentally appropriate approach to care delivery, one that was influenced by a multitude of initiatives such as a noise reduction program with music for babies dreaming, cot covers used on incubators to reduce noise and light, reduced fluorescent lighting above open cots, individualized care of each baby with cluster care to maximize sleep time, increased staff awareness of the needs of the families and families welcomed into the unit resulting in staff appearing less rushed and more approachable. There was also a change in focus to care being about the baby and the family, rather than to the staff themselves. These initiatives formed the basis of a developmental program, as advocated by Als (1986), which incorporates family-centered care and promotes bonding (Byers, 2003).

Environmental stressors impact on the growth and development of the baby, disrupt sleep and wake patterns, and negatively impact on family bonding (Brandon et al., 1999; Field, 1990; Graven et al., 1992). Once nursing staff were aware of the significant impact that the environment, and they themselves, had on the growing neonate, as well as on the family relationship, they were willing to review practice in order to make changes. This of course was not as easy as it sounds; attitudes and behaviors have been noted to be the greatest obstacles to reducing noise levels (Graven, 2000), whilst staff are more likely to respond to changes if they themselves are involved in the process of change (Bremmer et al., 2003). It has taken a concerted effort by a team of environmental advocates within the SCN to ensure adoption and sustainability of differing work practices. This team consists of several nursing staff who indicated an interest in environmental care as well as the unit manager and nurse educators. The work undertaken has had considerable influence on the SCN atmosphere and resultant impact for the baby, the family, and staff:

> it influences you . . . become more aware of things so you change the way you would normally do things . . . for instance about the noise in the isolette . . . bing bang everywhere . . . it is really a noxious environment . . . so when you have been educated . . . you keep the noise level down.

The noise of nursing interventions can result in the baby changing from a sleep state, to a fussy, crying state resulting in percentage oxygen saturation levels dropping to the low 80s (Zahr & Balian, 1995).

Simple things, like the introduction of cot covers, serve to reduce the impact of noise inside incubators (Saunders, 1995; Walsh-Sukys et al., 2001) and is therefore beneficial for the premature infant (Elander & Hellstrom, 1995; Robertson et al., 1999; Zahr & Balian, 1995). Furthermore, educating the team about how their behavior impacts on noise reduced noise levels (Bremmer et al., 2003):

> it makes such a big difference turning the lights off because you instantly walk in the door and it's dark and quiet and you tend to be dark and quiet, you don't talk as loud, it makes a huge difference.

Light has also been shown to stress neonates (Shogan & Schumann, 1993) and disrupt the sleep wake cycles (Brandon et al., 1999). Music also seems to help, since staff made a concerted effort to reduce noise levels in the unit as well as introducing *a lot more music that is suitable for babies rather than suitable for the nursing staff . . . nice gentle music is good for everyone . . . it calms us all.*

Family-centered care is widely promoted at a philosophical and policy levels within child healthcare (Brown & Ritchie, 1989; Caty et al., 2001; Darbyshire, 1994; Espezel & Canam, 2003; Franck & Callery, 2004; Hughes, 2007; Johnson & Lindschau, 1996; Lee, 2007; Maxton, 1997; Moore et al., 2003; Petersen et al., 2004; Tomlinson et al., 2002). The essence of care delivery is about questioning what we value about nursing and how we wish to participate in a meaningful process of care interaction. In order to develop this we must first describe what it is we are trying to achieve and then how we may achieve this in the messy reality of everyday practice.

> I think once you start getting involved . . . everybody just then . . . it becomes like a rippling, everybody goes with the flow, and there is not that mindset that blocking, and I think it works and people are then all working towards the same and enjoying and not dreading it.

Changing practice

These findings from the SCN give credence to the notion that successful change is enhanced when driven by those who implement care (Street, 1995); nurses are in the best position to ensure changes are sustained (Balfour & Clarke, 2001). The combined strategies used in this and other studies (Haffer, 1986) have been shown to be successful in facilitating practice change and the range of opportunities for engaging practitioner enhanced sustainability (Clarke et al., 1998). This has not only resulted in changes within the SCN but has reached other parts of the organization and impacted on practice changes elsewhere.

Evidence (such as research, practice guidelines, and policies) plays an important role in informing practice but this alone is not enough, as reflected in these examples. Nurses were often able to cite the research evidence about the environmental stressors of noise and light, but this did not result in consistent evidence-based practice. Thus, there needs to be an understanding of the context in which evidence is to be used and consideration given to exploring current practice (developing evidence about the culture itself) as this may provide the pathway for changing practice, as outlined here by Hooke et al. (2008, p. 89) reporting on a study about changing practice:

> The evidence was afforded greater value by virtue of the fact that, having been generated within that particular clinical context, it was indisputably part of the fabric of the ward's make-up. The ward could not be the same as it had been before the study because staff now knew things about themselves and their practice about which they had previously been unaware.

If we are to overcome the challenge of getting the evidence about family-centered care translated into everyday practice, we have to start from the point of enabling nursing staff to understand the context of their own practice and to question the difference between espoused ideals about practice (what we say we do) and the reality of such practice (what we actually do). In doing this we create a new evidence base about the context of practice, one that can be recognized and owned by those within that practice, providing the incentive to adopt evidence to inform ongoing care delivery.

Conclusion

This chapter has highlighted a number of important factors associated with the use of evidence in the pediatric healthcare context. The complexity of working with children and families has been explored through two key issues for pediatric practice, medication safety, and delivery of family-centered care, and uses research to explore the complexity of initiating practice change. It is clear that there is a plethora of evidence around these issues. It is not simply a case of presenting the evidence and hoping that it informs practice. Context and evidence are multifactorial. Staff do not work in isolation and their actions (or inactions) are influenced by the norms and rituals of the workplace, as well as by their knowledge of the research evidence. If evidence is to stand a chance of being successfully translated into practice there needs to be a critical review of existing work practices (behaviors, rituals, and assumptions) to identify contextual factors, plus consideration of the evidence, which in turn inform decisions about changes required. There is a need to review systems, processes, and the way people work, in light of the evidence about key issues such as medication safety, and then to work toward agreed changes in each of these areas so that we can achieve the desired outcomes. Using evidence to inform practice change is therefore fundamental to ensuring we provide the best possible care to children and their families.

References

Ahmad, T., Vickers, D., Campbell, S., Coulthard, M. & Pedler, S. (1991). Urine collection from disposable nappies. *Lancet*, 338, 674–676.

Ahmann, E. (1994). Family-centred care: Shifting orientation. *Pediatric Nursing*, 20, 113–116.

Als, H. (1986). A synactive model of neonatal behavioral organization: Framework for the assessment of neurobehavioral development in the premature infant and for support of parents in the intensive care environment. *Physical & Occupational Therapy in Pediatrics*, 6(3–4), 3–53.

Anderson, B. & Meakin, G. (2002). Scaling for size: Some implications for paediatric anaesthesia dosing. *Paediatric Anaesthesia*, 12(3), 205–219.

Baber, N. & Pritchard, D. (2003). Dose estimation for children. *British Journal of Clinical Pharmacology*, 56(5), 489–493.

Balfour, M. & Clarke, C. (2001). Searching for sustainable change. *Journal of Clinical Nursing*, 10, 44–50.

Bonati, N., Choonara, I., Hoppu, K., Pons, G. & Seyberth, H. (1999). Closing the gap in drug therapy. *Lancet*, 353(9164), 1625.

Bowie, B., Hall, R., Faulkner, J. & Anderson, B. (2003). Single-room infant care: Future trends in special care nursery planning and design. *Neonatal Network*, 22, 27–34.

Bradley, S. (1996). Processes in the creation and diffusion of nursing knowledge: An examination of the developing concept of family-centred care. *Journal of Advanced Nursing*, 23, 722–727.

Bradley, C.F. & Wiggins, S. (1983). An evaluation of family-centered maternity care. *Women & Health*, 8(1), 35–47.

Brandon, D., Holditch-Davis, D. & Belyea, M. (1999). Nursing care and the development of sleeping and waking behaviors in preterm infants. *Research in Nursing and Health*, 22, 217–229.

Bratt, M., Broome, M., Kelber, S. & Lostocco, L. (2000). Influence of stress and nursing leadership on job satisfaction of pediatric intensive care nurses. *American Journal of Critical Care*, 18, 79–86.

Bremmer, P., Byers, J. & Kiehl, E. (2003). Noise and the premature infant: Physiological effects and practice implications. *Journal of Obstetric, Gynecologic, and Neonatal Nursing*, 32, 447–454.

Brown, J. & Ritchie, J. (1989). Nurses' perceptions of their relationship with parents. *Maternal-Child Nursing Journal*, 18, 79–86.

Bruce, B. & Ritchie, J. (1997). Nurses' practices and perceptions of family-centred care. *Journal of Pediatric Nursing*, 12, 214–221.

Byers, J. (2003). Care and the evidence for their use in the NICU. *American Journal of Maternal Child Nursing*, 28, 174–180.

Callery, P. & Smith, L. (1991). A study of role negotiation between nurses and the parents of hospitalised children. *Journal of Advanced Nursing*, 17, 772–781.

Casey, A. (1995). Partnership nursing: Influences on involvement of informal carers. *Journal of Advanced Nursing*, 22, 1058–1062.

Catlett, A. & Holditch-Davis, D. (1990). Environmental stimulation of the acutely ill premature infant. Physiological effects and nursing implications. *Neonatal Network*, 8, 19–25.

Caty, S., Larocque, S. & Koren, I. (2001). Family-centered care in Ontario general hospitals: The views of pediatric nurses. *Canadian Journal of Nursing Leadership*, 14, 10–18.

Chapell, K. & Newman, C. (2004). Potential tenfold drug overdoses on a neonatal unit. *Archives of Diseases in Childhood. Fetal and Neonatal Edition*, 89, F483–F484.

Clark, A. & Carter, P. (2002). Why do nurses see families as "trouble?" *Clinical Nurse Specialist*, 16, 40–41.

Clarke, C., Procter, S. & Watson, B. (1998). Making changes: A survey to identify mediators in the development of health care practice. *Clinical Effectiveness in Nursing*, 2, 30–36.

Cohen, H. (1997). Urine samples for disposable diapers: An accurate method for urine culture. *The Journal of Family Practice*, 44, 290–292.

Conroy, S., Choonara, I., Impicciatore, P. et al. (2000). Survey of unlicensed and off-label drugs use in paediatric wards in European countries. *British Medical Journal*, 320, 79–82.

Cox, B. (1974). Rooming in. *Nursing Times*, 17, 1246–1247.

Coyne, I. (1996). Parent participation: A concept analysis. *Journal of Advanced Nursing*, 23, 733–740.

Coyne, I. & Cowley, S. (2007). Challenging the philosophy of partnership with parents: A grounded theory study. *International Journal of Nursing Studies*, 44, 893–904.

Daneman, S., Macaluso, J. & Guzzetta, C. (2003). Healthcare providers' attitudes towards parent participation in the care of the hospitalized child. *Journal for Specialist Pediatric Nursing, 8,* 90–98.

Darbyshire, P. (1994). *Living with a Sick Child in Hospital. The Experiences of Parents and Nurses.* London: Chapman & Hall.

Davis, L., Edwards, H., Mohay, H. & Wollin, J. (2003). The impact of very premature birth on the psychological health of mothers. *Early Human Development, 73,* 61–70.

Eckle, N. & MacLean, S. (2001). Assessment of family-centred care policies and practices for pediatric patients in nine US emergency departments. *Journal of Emergency Nursing, 27,* 238–245.

Elander, G. & Hellstrom, G. (1995). Reduction of noise levels in intensive care units for infants: Evaluation of an intervention program. *Heart & Lung: The Journal of Critical Care, 24,* 376–379.

Espezel, H. & Canam, C. (2003). Parent–nurse interactions: Care of hospitalized children. *Journal of Advanced Nursing, 44,* 34–41.

Fegran L., Fagermoen, M.S. & Helseth, S. (2008). Development of parent–nurse relationships in neonatal intensive care units—from closeness to detachment. *Journal of Advanced Nursing, 64,* 363–371.

Fenwick, J., Barclay, L. & Schmied, V. (1999). Activities and interactions in Level II nurseries: A report of an ethnographic study. *Journal of Perinatal and Neonatal Nursing, 13,* 53–65.

Fenwick, J., Barclay, L. & Schmied, V. (2001). "Chatting": An important clinical tool in facilitating mothering in neonatal nurseries. *Journal of Advanced Nursing, 33,* 583–593.

Field, T. (1990). Alleviating stress in newborn infants in the intensive care unit. *Clinics in Perinatology, 17,* 1–9.

Fisher, C., Lindhorst, H., Matthews, T., Munroe, D., Paulin, D. & Scott, D. (2008). Nursing staff attitudes and behaviours regarding family presence in the hospital setting. *Journal of Advanced Nursing, 64,* 615–624.

Fisher, H. (2001). The needs of parents with chronically sick children: A literature review. *Journal of Advanced Nursing, 36,* 600–607.

Fortescue, E., Kaushal, R., Landrigan, C. et al. (2003). Prioritizing strategies for preventing medication errors and adverse drug events in pediatric inpatients. *Pediatrics, 111,* 722–729.

Franck, L. & Callery, P. (2004). Re-thinking family centred care across the continuum of children's healthcare. *Child: Care, Health and Development, 30,* 265–277.

Ghaleb, M. & Wong, I. (2006). Medication errors in paediatric patients. *Archives of Disease in Childhood – Education and Practice, 91,* 20–24.

Gill, K. (1987). Parents participation with a family health focus: Nurses' attitudes. *Pediatric Nursing, 13,* 94–96.

Gordin, P. and Johnson, B. (1999). Technology and family-centred perinatal care: Conflict or synergy? *Journal of Obstetric, Gynecologic, and Neonatal Nursing, 28,* 401–408.

Graven, S. (2000). Sound and the developing infant in the NICU: Conclusions and recommendations for care. *Journal of Perinatology*, 20, 88–93.

Graven, S., Bowen, F., Brooten, D. et al. (1992). The high-risk infant environment. Part 1: The role of the neonatal intensive care unit in the outcome of high-risk infants. *Journal of Perinatology*, 12, 164–172.

Haffer, A. (1986). Facilitating change. Choosing the appropriate strategy. *Journal of Nursing Administration*, 16, 18–22.

Hart, D. (1979). Parents and professionals as partners. *New Horizons in Education*, 61, 8–11.

Harvey, G., Loftus-Hills, A., Rycroft-Malone, J. et al. (2002). Getting evidence into practice: The role and function of facilitation. *Journal of Advanced Nursing*, 37(6), 577–588.

Hicks, R., Becker, S. & Chuo, J. (2007a). A summary of NICU fat emulsion medication errors and nursing services: Data from MEDMARX. *Advances in Neonatal Care*, 7(6), 299–308.

Hicks, R., Becker, S., Windle, P. & Krenzischek, D. (2007b). Medication errors in the PACU. *Journal of Perianesthesia Nursing*, 22(6), 413–419.

Hooke, N., Lewis, P., Kelly, M., Wilson, V. & Jones, S. (2008). Making something of it: One ward's application of evidence into practice. *Practice Development in Health Care*, 7(2), 79–91.

Hughes, M. (2007). Parents' and nurses' attitudes to family-centred care: An Irish perspective. *Journal of Clinical Nursing*, 16, 2341–2348.

Hughes, R. & Edgerton, E. (2005). First, do no harm: Reducing pediatric medication errors. *The American Journal of Nursing*, 105(5), 79–84.

Hutchfield, K. (1999). Family-centred care: A concept analysis. *Journal of Advanced Nursing*, 29, 1178–1187.

Johnson, A. & Lindschau, A. (1996). Staff attitudes toward parent participation in the care of children who are hospitalized. *Pediatric Nursing*, 22, 99–102, 120.

Johnson, B., Jeppson, E. & Redburn, L. (1992). *Caring for Children and Families: Guidelines for Hospitals*. Bethesda, MD: Association for the Care of Children's Health.

Keatinge, D. & Gilmore, V. (1996). Shared care: A partnership between parents and nurses. *Australian Journal of Advanced Nursing*, 14, 28–36.

Knight, L. (1995). Negotiating care roles. *Nursing Times*, 91, 31–33.

Koppel, R., Wetterneck, T., Tilles, J. & Karsh, B.-T. (2008). Workarounds to barcode medication administration systems: Their occurrences, causes, and threats to patient safety. *Journal of the American Informatics Association*, 15, 408–423.

Kozer, E. (2009). Medication errors in children. *Paediatric Drugs*, 11(1), 52–54.

Kozer, E., Scolnik, D., Jarvis, A. & Koren, G. (2006). The effect of detection approaches on the reported incidence of tenfold errors. *Drug Safety*, 29(2), 169–174.

Lee, P. (2007). What does partnership in care mean for children's nurses? *Journal of Clinical Nursing*, 16, 518–526.

Lightbody, T. (2009). The importance of family-centred care in the NICU. *Canadian Nurse*, 105, 11–12.

Lotas, M. (1992). Effects of light and sound in the neonatal intensive care unit environment on the low-birthweight infant. *NAACOG's Clinical Issues in Perinatal and Women's Health Nursing*, 3, 34–44.

Maxton, F. (1997). Old habits die hard: Changing paediatric nurses' perceptions of families in ICU. *Intensive & Critical Care Nursing*, 13, 145–150.

Moore, K., Coker, K., DuBuisson, A., Swett, B. & Edwards, W. (2003). Implementing potentially better practices for improving family-centered care in neonatal intensive care units: Successes and challenges. *Pediatrics*, 111, 450–460.

McCaughan, D., Thompson, C., Cullum, N., Sheldon, T. & Thompson, D. (2002). Acute care nurses' perceptions of barriers to using research information in clinical decision making. *Journal of Advanced Nursing*, 39, 46–60.

McGrath, J. (2000). Developmentally supportive caregiving and technology in the NICU: Isolation or merger of intervention strategies? *Journal of Perinatal and Neonatal Nursing*, 14, 78–91.

McGrath, J. (2001). Building relationships with families in the NICU: Exploring the guarded alliance. *Journal of Perinatal and Neonatal Nursing*, 15, 74–83.

McKune, I. (1989). Catch or bag specimen? *Nursing Times*, 85(37), 80–82.

McPhillips, H., Stille, C., Smith, D. et al. (2005). Potential medication dosing errors in outpatient pediatrics. *Journal of Pediatrics*, 147, 761–767.

National Collaborating Centre for Women's and Children's Health (2007). Urinary tract infection in children: Diagnosis, treatment and long-term management. London, UK: National Institute for Health and Clinical Excellence. Available at http://guidance.nice.org.uk/CG54.

Newman, M., Papadopoulos, I. & Sigsworth, J. (1998). Barriers to evidence-based practice. *Intensive & Critical Care Nursing*, 14, 231–238.

Newton, M. (2000). Family-centered care: Current realities in parent participation. *Pediatric Nursing*, 26, 164–168.

Nichols, P., Copeland, T.-S., Craib, I., Hopkins, P. & Bruce, D. (2008). Learning from error: Identifying contributory causes of medication errors in an Australian hospital. *Medical Journal of Australia*, 188, 276–279.

O'Connor, J., Vietze, P., Sherrod, K., Sandler, H. & Altemeier, W. (1980). Reducing incidence of parental inadequacy following rooming in. *Pediatrics*, 66, 176–182.

Paavilainen, E. & Astedt-Kurkl, P. (1997). The client–nurse relationship as experienced by public health nurses: Towards better collaboration. *Public Health Nursing*, 14, 137–142.

Perkins, E., Ginn, L., Fanning, J. & Bartlett, D. (2004). Effect of nursing education on positioning of infants in the neonatal intensive care unit. *Pediatric Physical Therapy*, 16, 2–12.

Petersen, M., Cohen, J. & Parson, V. (2004). Family-centred care: Do we practice what we preach? *Journal of Obstetric Gynecologic and Neonatal Nursing*, 33, 421–427.

Power, N. & Franck, L. (2008). Parent participation in the care of hospitalized children: A systematic review. *Journal of Advanced Nursing*, 62, 622–641.

Prot, S., Fontan, J., Alberti, C. et al. (2005). Drug administration errors and their determinants in pediatric in-patients. *International Journal for Quality in Health Care*, 17, 381–389.

Ramos, M. (1992). The nurse patient relationship: Themes and variations. *Journal of Advanced Nursing*, 17, 496–506.

Reason, J. (2000). Human error: Models and management. *British Medical Journal*, 320, 768–770.

Retsas, A. (2000). Barriers to using research evidence in nursing practice. *Journal of Advanced Nursing*, 31, 599–606.

Robertson, A., Cooper-Peel, C. & Vos, P. (1999). Contribution of heating, ventilation, air conditioning airflow and conversation to the ambient sound in the neonatal intensive care unit. *Journal of Perinatology*, 19, 362–366.

Robinson, L. (2003). An organisational guide for an effective developmental program in the NICU. *Journal of Obstetric Gynaecological and Neonatal Nursing*, 32, 379–386.

Rowe, J. & Jones, L. (2008). Facilitating transitions. Nursing support for parents during the transfer of preterm infants between neonatal nurseries. *Journal of Clinical Nursing*, 17, 782–789.

Rushton, C. & Glover, J. (1990). Involving parents in decisions to forego life-sustaining treatment for critically ill infants and children. *American Association of Critical-Care Nurses: Clinical Issues in Critical Care Nursing*, 1, 206–214.

Rycroft-Malone, J. (2004a). Research implementation: Evidence, context and facilitation—the PARIHS framework. In: McCormack, B., Manley, K. & Garbett, R. (eds) *Practice Development in Nursing*. Oxford: Blackwell.

Rycroft-Malone, J. (2004b). The PARIHS framework—a framework for guiding the implementation of evidence-based practice. *Journal of Nursing Care Quality*, 19, 297–304.

Rycroft-Malone, J., Harvey, G., Kitson, A., McCormack, B., Seers, K. & Titchen, A. (2002). Getting evidence into practice: Ingredients for change. *Nursing Standard*, 16(37), 38–43.

Sams, L., Penn, B. & Facteau, L. (2004). The challenge of using evidence-based practice. *Journal of Nursing Administration*, 34(9), 407–414.

Saunders, A. (1995). Incubator noise: A method to decrease decibels. *Pediatric Nursing*, 21, 265–268.

Shelton, T., Jeppson, E. & Johnson, B. (1987). *Family-centred care for children with special health care needs*. Bethesda, MD: Association for the Care of Children's Health.

Shogan, M. & Schumann, L. (1993). The effect of environmental lighting on the oxygen saturation of preterm infants in the NICU. *Neonatal Network*, 12, 7–13.

Sinha, Y. & Cranswick, N. (2007). Prescribing safely for children. *Journal of Paediatrics & Child Health*, 43,112–116.

Smith, F. (1995). *Children's Nursing in Practice: Nottingham Model.* Oxford: Blackwell Science.

Smith, S., Lewis, P. & Wilson, V. (2009). A "wee" problem: Using action research to facilitate a change in urine collection methods. *Neonatal, Paediatric and Child Health Nursing*, 12, 15–19.

Stephenson, T. (2005). The National Patient Safety Agency. *Archives of Disease in Childhood*, 90, 226–228.

Street, A. (1995). *Nursing Replay: Researching Nursing Culture Together.* Melbourne: Churchill Livingstone.

Taylor, J., Loan, L., Kamara, J., Blackburn, S. & Whitney, D. (2008). Medication administration variances before and after implementation of computerized physician order entry in a neonatal intensive care unit. *Pediatrics*, 121,123–128.

Thompson, C., McCaughan, D., Cullum, N., Sheldon, T., Mulhall, A. & Thompson, D. (2001). Research information and nurses' clinical decision making: What is useful. *Journal of Advanced Nursing*, 36, 376–388.

Tomlinson, P., Thomlinson, E., Peden-McAlipine, C. & Kirschabaum, M. (2002). Clinical innovation for promoting family care in pediatric intensive care: Demonstration, role modelling and reflective practice. *Journal of Advanced Nursing*, 38, 161–170.

Turner, S., Nunn, A., Fielding, K. & Choonara, I. (1999). Adverse drug reactions to unlicensed and off label drugs on paediatric wards: A prospective study. *Acta Paediatrica*, 88, 965–968.

Trnobranski, P. (1994). Nurse–patient negotiation: Assumption or reality? *Journal of Advanced Nursing*, 19, 733–737.

Van Riper, M. (2001). Family-provider relationships and well-being in families with preterm infants in NICU. *Heart & Lung: The Journal of Critical Care*, 30, 74–84.

Waddington, P. & Watson, A. (1997). Which urine collection bag? *Paediatric Nursing*, 9(2), 19–20.

Walsh, K., Kaushal, R. & Chessare, J. (2005). How to avoid paediatric medication errors: A user's guide to the literature. *Archives of Disease in Childhood*, 90, 698–702.

Walsh, K., Landrigan, C., Adams, W. et al. (2008). Effect of computer order entry on prevention of serious medication errors in hospitalized children. *Pediatrics*, 121, 421–427.

Walsh-Sukys, M., Reitenbach, M., Hudson-Barr, K. & Depompei, P. (2001). Reducing light and sound in the neonatal intensive care unit: An evaluation of patient safety, staff satisfaction and costs. *Journal of Perinatology*, 21, 230–235.

WHO (2007). Make medicines child size. Available at www.who.int/childmedicines/en (accessed October 22, 2009).

Wilson, V. (2005). Developing a culture of family centred care: An emancipatory practice development approach. Unpublished PhD Thesis, Monash University, Melbourne.

Wilson, V., McCormack, B. & Ives, G. (2005). Understanding the workplace culture of a special care nursery. *Journal of Advanced Nursing*, 50, 27–38.

Wong, E., Taylor, Z., Thompson, J. & Tuthill, D. (2009a). A simplified gentamicin dosing chart is quicker and more accurate for nurse verification than the BNFc. *Archives of Disease in Childhood*, 94, 542–545.

Wong, I., Wong, L. & Cranswick, N. (2009b). Minimising medication errors in children. *Archives of Disease in Childhood*, 94, 161–164.

Zahr, L. & Balian, S. (1995). Responses of premature infants to routine nursing interventions and noise in the NICU. *Nursing Research*, 44, 179–185.

Chapter 6

Making context work in the perioperative setting

Victoria M. Steelman

Introduction

The perioperative setting presents a high-risk context for patient care with unique challenges for evidence-based practice. The context involves the patient, the environment and technology, and human factors of the surgical team. Patients come to the operating room with a host of predisposing factors that influence their outcomes. These may include risk factors for surgical site infection (e.g., diabetes, low serum albumin, and existing infection) or injury (e.g., impaired circulation, preoperative hypothermia, and morbid obesity). Once in the operating room, anesthesia, surgical interventions, technology, and prolonged immobilization may contribute to the potential for infection or injury. Human factors, including the rapid pace, challenges with communication, and multitasking all add to the context of a very high-risk experience for the patient.

To minimize these risks, perioperative nurses have traditionally implemented a host of policies and procedures based upon their collective experiences and consensus. Some of these practices are designed to minimize the risk of surgical site infection by reducing microbial contamination of the surgical site (e.g., environmental cleaning, operating room attire, aseptic technique, and sterilization). Other practices focus on safe use of high-risk equipment (e.g., electrosurgery, lasers, and tourniquets). And other practices are designed to minimize the risk of injury from anesthesia (e.g., preoperative fasting), positioning (e.g., padding of bony prominences and nerves), and the surgical intervention (e.g., counting surgical sponges).

Until recently, evidence-based practice has not significantly influenced this perioperative patient care, because of the limited amount of high-level evidence available. There are very few randomized clinical trials that examine the effects of traditional practices on patient outcomes. Moreover, it would be unethical to conduct much of this research. For example, there is no published research to indicate that it is necessary to sterilize surgical instruments. Yet, this practice has become the standard of care. It would be unethical to randomly assign patients to receive surgery using unsterilized instruments. The same is true when studying other practices that have become the standard of care for prevention of surgical site infection and patient injury. A second challenge is the complexity of studying surgical site infection. There are many factors contributing to the development of a surgical site infection, including predisposing factors of the patient, the microorganism, and factors associated with the procedure, patient care, and environment. Some of these factors cannot be adequately measured and others cannot be controlled. To study factors that can be measured would require a research design with a very large sample size and adequate control over contributing factors. This type of research is exceptionally difficult and expensive to do. So, much of what we would like to know about prevention of surgical site infections remains unanswered by high-level evidence. In the past, this resulted in limited interest in the application of research findings in perioperative care.

This paradigm has shifted in recent years. In 1999, the U.S. Centers for Disease Control and Prevention published a sentinel systematic review and recommendations for prevention of surgical site infection (Mangram et al., 1999). In the past few years, international groups have accepted the challenge of implementing these recommendations. One of these groups is the Surgical Care Improvement Project (SCIP). The SCIP's goal is to reduce the incidence of surgical complications nationally by 25% by the year 2010 by implementing key evidence-based practices in hospitals (Table 6.1).

The term "evidence-based practice" has become somewhat of a cliché in perioperative nursing, with many misconceptions about what level of evidence is required to implement changes in perioperative practice. Some would argue that evidence-based practice requires multiple-site randomized controlled trials. Others support

Table 6.1 Surgical care improvement project core measures*

- Surgery patients on a beta-blocker prior to arrival that received a beta-blocker during the perioperative period.
- Prophylactic antibiotic received within one hour prior to surgical incision.
- Prophylactic antibiotic selection for surgical patients.
- Prophylactic antibiotics discontinued within 24 hours after surgery end time (48 hours for cardiac patients).
- Cardiac surgery patients with controlled 6 a.m. postoperative serum glucose.
- Surgery patients with appropriate hair removal.
- Colorectal surgery patients with immediate postoperative normothermia.

*Surgical Care Improvement Project. Available at http://www.qualitynet.org/dcs/ContentServer?level 3=Measures&c=MQParents&pagename=Medqic%2FMeasure%2FMeasuresHome&cid=1137346750659& parentName=TopicCat (accessed August 15, 2009).

lower levels of evidence. For the purposes of this chapter, evidence-based practice is considered in the broader context of using the best evidence available to make decisions that direct patient care. It is a philosophy of professional life that enables us to achieve excellence individually and as a professional nursing specialty. This high-level decision-making process provides the power to drive change in a complex, interdisciplinary, cost-conscious healthcare arena.

Within the context of the operating room, nurses should base patient care on a balance of knowledge gained through research findings, known risks, and professional experience.

In the presence of known risks to the patient, decisions must be made that appropriately support positive patient outcomes. How to do this when high-level evidence is limited poses a challenge that can be addressed through a decision-making model using the best evidence that is available.

Within this model, the hierarchy starts with the highest level of evidence, and progresses down through lower levels of evidence. The significant difference in this hierarchy from others is the inclusion of these lower levels of evidence (Figure 6.1).

Meta-analyses

Meta-analyses are the strongest evidence to guide practice. Meta-analyses published in the Cochrane Collaboration's library can be

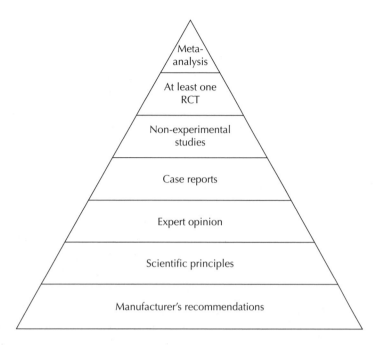

Figure 6.1 Hierarchy of evidence used in the perioperative setting.

used to minimize the risk of complication, reduce cost and eliminate unnecessary work, and reduce the risk of personnel injury. Four examples highlighted here that are highly relevant to perioperative practice include (a) preoperative fasting, (b) thromboembolism prevention, (c) bowel preps, and (d) double gloving.

Preoperative fasting

Traditionally, surgical patients have been prohibited from receiving fluids and food after midnight on the day of surgery. The rationale used was that this would minimize the risk of aspiration; however, this practice causes discomfort for the patient and has been questioned. Evidence was assembled and evaluated in a systematic review and meta-analysis for the Cochrane Collaboration (Brady et al., 2003). These researchers included 38 randomized controlled comparisons, primarily healthy adults. Subjects who drank water had less gastric volume than those fasting. The researchers concluded that there is no evidence that a shortened fasting time increases the risk of aspiration, regurgitation, or related morbidity. These findings supported the work of the American Society of Anesthesiologists in their clinical practice guideline (American Society of Anesthesiologists Task Force on Preoperative Fasting, 1999). In 2005, the UK's Royal College of Nursing built further on the meta-analyses and developed a clinical practice guideline for perioperative fasting in adults and children (RCN, 2005). Thus perioperative nurses should incorporate this evidence into patient education and protocols for surgical preparation.

Thromoembolism prevention

Prolonged immobilization in surgery can result in thromboembolism, a potentially life-threatening complication. Perioperative nurses sometimes wonder about the best way to prevent this complication, and might not fully appreciate the value of combined modalities. Wille-Jørgensen et al. (2004) conducted a meta-analysis of 19 studies of general surgery patients, including subjects undergoing colon surgery. Three therapies were evaluated: (1) unfractionated heparin (LDH), (2) low-molecular weight heparin (LMWH), and (3) mechanical compression. The outcomes measured included deep vein thrombosis (DVT) and pulmonary emboli (PE). Heparins were found to be better than a placebo at preventing DVTs and PEs (odds ratio 0.32), and LDH and LMWH were found equally effective (odds ratio 1.01). The combination of graded compression stockings and LDH was found to be better than LDH alone in preventing DVT and/or PE (odds ratio 4.17). There were insufficient data to compare the use of pneumatic compression stockings versus graduated compression stockings or the use of either of these devices against no treatment or prophylaxis with heparin. The authors concluded that the optimal prophylaxis for colorectal surgery is the combination of graduated compression stockings and LDH or LMWH. Additional evidence to aid decision making comes in the form of the Clinical Guideline CG92, issued by the National Institute for Health and Clinical Excellence (NICE) in January 2010; for further details go to http://guidance.nice.org.uk/CG92/Guidance/pdf/English and quick reference guide http://guidance.nice.org.uk/CG92/QuickRefGuide/pdf/English.

Perioperative nurses should participate in the prevention of DVTs and PEs by applying the compression stockings, verifying that they properly fit, and assuring that any prescribed heparin is administered preoperatively.

Mechanical bowel preparation before colon surgery

Mechanical bowel preparation has traditionally been performed to minimize contamination of the surgical site and reduce the risk of surgical site infection. However, these procedures are time consuming, expensive, and very unpleasant for the patient. Patients undergoing elective colon surgery are usually admitted the morning of surgery; the need for bowel preps upon patient arrival can also lead to a delay in the surgery. This practice was questioned and addressed through a meta-analysis (Guenaga et al., 2009). An analysis of 14 randomized clinical trials found no significant differences between groups receiving bowel preparation and receiving no preparation when evaluating patient outcomes (anastomotic leakage, wound infection, peritonitis, need for reoperation, non-abdominal complications, and mortality rates). This meta-analysis is strong evidence that the use of preoperative mechanical bowel preparation can be discontinued as a sacred cow, eliminating the patient discomfort, cost, and potential surgical delays. It provides newer evidence than was reviewed for the CDC Guideline on Prevention of Surgical Site Infection (Mangram et al., 1999), and highlights the importance of reviewing current evidence when reviewing clinical practice guidelines. Perioperative nurses should collaborate with surgeons to determine the best application of this evidence in the clinical setting.

Double gloving to prevent sharps injuries

Needlestick and sharps injuries are a serious hazard exposing healthcare workers to blood-borne pathogens. In the operating room, gloves have traditionally been worn to protect the patient from microorganisms on the hands of the surgical team members, but also serve as a barrier to the transmission of blood-borne pathogens from the patient to the clinician. A single pair of gloves is often not an adequate barrier. Glove failures occur frequently during operations. Most (83 %) of these glove perforations are undetected during procedures (Thomas et al., 2001).

A systematic review and meta-analysis was undertaken to evaluate the utility of double gloving (Tanner & Parkinson, 2006). Nine randomized clinical trials were found acceptable for inclusion. Results of this analysis demonstrated that:

- perforation rates are similar for the outer glove when double gloving, compared to single gloves ($p = 0.3$)

- there are significantly fewer perforations to the inner glove when double gloving, compared to single gloves ($p < 0.00001$)
- more outer glove perforations are detected when using a colored underglove compared to wearing two pairs of standard latex gloves ($p = 0.002$).

Therefore, double gloving can prevent exposures that could lead to transmission of blood-borne pathogens to the surgical team and reduce the cost of these exposure workups. Stebral and Steelman (2006) implemented this evidence-based practice as a recommendation in clinical practice. Even with modest adherence to the change, they found a 23.5% reduction in sharps injuries.

Randomized clinical trials

Randomized clinical trials are considered to be a very high level of evidence, and have often been referred to as the gold standard for evidence-based practice. This has been challenged (Grossman & Mackenzie, 2005) and often more than one clinical trial, or a combination of randomized clinical trials and lower levels of evidence is needed to address the complexity of perioperative interventions.

Preoperative showers

Preoperative bathing or showering before surgery has been an accepted practice for decades. This mechanical cleansing removes transient and resident flora from the patient's skin. The Centers for Disease Control and Prevention recommendation is to "require patients to shower or bathe with an antiseptic agent at least the night before the operative day. *Category IB*" (Mangram et al., 1999). Pottinger et al. (2006) reviewed seven clinical trials (five randomized, one non-randomized, one prospective cross-over) to determine the effectiveness of this intervention. The methods included one to three bath/showers with an antimicrobial agent (4% chlorhexidine gluconate [CHG], povidone [PVP]–iodine, or soap [medicated, non-medicated, or soap with lotion]). The outcome measured was bacterial colony counts in four studies and surgical site infection rates in three studies.

This systematic review of the research supports the use of preoperative showers to reduce bacterial counts on the skin. The most effective agent was CHG, and more than one shower is necessary to achieve maximum antimicrobial activity. However, the research does not definitively link this decrease in microbial skin count with a reduction in surgical site infection rates. This link remains theoretical.

Although preoperative showers or bathing has been recommended for many years, the actual practice has changed with the transition to outpatient surgery. This evidence supports the need to instruct patients to perform two showers with CHG. Unfortunately the best strategy for maximizing compliance is unknown. Research is needed to determine if providing patients with the antiseptic enhances compliance and which teaching methodology is most effective.

Prevention of perioperative hypothermia

Unplanned hypothermia is among the most common complications of surgery. Anesthesia impairs thermoregulation, which is coupled with the heat loss from the incision and exposed skin into the surgical environment. A randomized clinical trial was used to evaluate the effect of hypothermia on the risk of surgical site infection: 19% of hypothermic subjects developed surgical site infection, compared with 6% who remained normothermic (Kurz et al., 1996). These findings were supported by a non-randomized, prospective cohort study (Flores-Maldonado et al., 2001). Coupled with a non-randomized study linking hypothermia to adverse cardiac events (including ventricular tachycardia) (Frank et al., 1993) and another linking hypothermia with increased blood loss (Flores-Maldonado et al., 1997), the combined evidence provides strong rationale to implement measures to prevent perioperative hypothermia.

Forced-air warming is a safe and the widely used active warming method in the perioperative setting. The efficacy of forced-air warming in preventing unplanned hypothermia has been proven in many clinical trials. It is more effective than reflection insulation (Borms et al., 1994; Ng et al., 2003) circulating fluid mattresses, a radiant heat lamp (Murat et al., 1994), or warmed blankets (Mason et al., 1998; Ng et al., 2003).

One of the challenges with prevention of hypothermia occurs when the patient is hypothermic preoperatively. This can result from major trauma, burns, hypothyroidism, hypopituitarism, or in neonates. Perioperative nurses should assess the temperature of patients preoperatively, and ensure that the warming is initiated preoperatively. Fossum et al. (2001) studied the use of preoperative warming with forced-air warming. Patients receiving the intervention preoperatively had significantly higher temperatures than patients receiving warmed cotton blankets (Box 6.1).

Perioperative nurses should use forced-air warming for all surgical patients undergoing anesthesia for more than 1 h. More research is needed to determine the most effective duration of time to administer

---

Box 6.1 A comparison study on the effects of prewarming patients in the outpatient surgery setting*

Purpose: The primary purpose of this study was to determine if there was a difference in core body temperature upon arrival in the postanesthesia care unit (PACU) between patients who were warmed preoperatively with a forced warm air blanket and those patients warmed with cotton blankets.

Sample: The sample was 100 adult patients undergoing gynecological, orthopedic, or urologic procedures under general anesthesia for 1–3 h. All subjects had an American Society of Anesthesiologists acuity rating or I, II, or III.

Methods: Subjects were randomly assigned to an experimental group receiving prewarming by using forced-air warming ($n = 50$) or a control group receiving prewarming with cotton blankets preheated in an electric blanket warmer set at 66°C ($n = 50$). Temperatures were monitored every 15 min preoperatively and postoperatively.

Results: Patients in the forced-air warming group had significantly higher temperatures upon arrival in the PACU than did patients in the warm blanket group ($p = 0.000$). Patients in the forced-air warming group exhibited a very slight increase in temperature of 0.0067°C (±0.52) compared with a decrease in temperature of 0.22°C (±0.48) for patients in the control group.

Conclusion: Preoperative warming with warmed cotton blankets is not as effective as using forced-air warming for maintaining core body temperature perioperatively. Warmed cotton blankets should be considered a comfort measure only.

---

*Fossum et al. (2001).

forced-air warming preoperatively in order to achieve the best outcomes.

Non-experimental studies

Other types of research provide compelling evidence to guide perioperative patient care and identify the gaps requiring further research. Epidemiologic studies can determine the incidence of a problem and relationships between variables that cannot be ethically studied through randomized clinical trials. For example, when we want to know the incidence of adverse events and risk factors that contribute to these events, non-experimental studies are very valuable.

Case–control studies

Retained swabs/sponges and other foreign bodies after surgery is a very serious adverse event. Prevention of these medical errors is an important part of the perioperative nurse's work. Patient safety organizations have dubbed these as "never events," indicating that they should never occur (U.S. HHS, 2006). Gawande et al. (2003) studied the patient outcomes and risk factors for retained sponges. The outcomes to the patient are very serious, including:

- reoperation (69%)
- readmission or prolonged length of stay (43%)
- sepsis or infection (43%)
- fistula or bowel obstruction (15%)
- visceral perforation (7%)
- death (2%).

Using a retrospective case–control study design, these researchers found that some factors increased the risk of retained sponge, including:

- emergency surgery
- unplanned change in the operation
- higher body mass index (Gawande et al., 2003).

The primary strategy used to prevent retained sponges and instruments is counting these surgical supplies before the procedure and twice when closing the incision. Researchers studying this practice found that count discrepancies identified 77% and prevented 54% of retained items. The rate of retained items was 1 in 70 with a count discrepancy, and discrepancies increase with:

- duration of the surgery
- late time procedures
- number of nursing teams (Egorova et al., 2008).

We know from this non-experimental research that when a sponge is retained, it can lead to serious patient outcomes. Attention to detail when handling counted items is critical. But more research is needed to evaluate strategies for prevention and work toward a fail-safe method of prevention.

Outbreak investigations

Valuable information can also be gained through epidemiologic surveillance and outbreak investigations. A recent example involves an investigation of *Pseudomonas aeruginosa* infections following bronchoscopy (DiazGranados et al., 2009). A cross-sectional study was undertaken to determine if a cluster of infections was associated with a specific bronchoscope. Twelve patients cultured positive for a unique susceptibility strain of *P. aeruginosa*; 55% of patients receiving a specific bronchoscope cultured positive for the organism. Investigators cultured the bronchoscope after high-level disinfection and found that the culture was positive with the same unique strain of *P. aeruginosa*. An engineering evaluation was undertaken and multiple defects were found, presumed to be caused by damage during repeated uses. The bronchoscope had passed the visual inspection and leak testing routinely performed during reprocessing. However, it had not been sent in for preventive maintenance as recommended by the manufacturer. This routine engineering evaluation would, in all likelihood, have identified these defects. This study highlights the risks inherent with complex medical devices that are difficult to clean and disinfect or sterilize. Routine preventive maintenance is a very important quality control measure that should be scheduled according to the manufacturers' instructions.

Germain et al. (2005) described a cluster of transmissions of hepatitis C from patient to patient in the operating room. The cause was techniques associated with multidose vials for medications administered by one anesthesia provider. The same syringe was used to withdraw fentanyl citrate multiple times and inject into the lines of different patients. Use of a common syringe for multiple patients or reinsertion of a used needle into a multidose vial is a breach of infection control practices. This study heightens our awareness of the risks associated with this practice. Pressure for shortened times between cases should not trigger healthcare providers to take unsafe shortcuts.

Failure Modes and Effects Analysis

Another type of evidence that is very valuable to understanding the risks associated with perioperative care is a hazard or risk assessment. These methods have been borrowed from manufacturing industries. One type of risk assessment, used by the Institute for Healthcare Improvement (IHI), is the Failure Modes and Effects Analysis (FMEA). FMEA is a systematic, proactive method for evaluating a process to identify where and how it might fail, and to assess the relative impact of different failures. This methodology can be used for designing preventive strategies focusing on the steps of the process recognized as posing the highest risk. This process has been used to identify the potential failures when implementing programmable intravenous pumps (Wetterneck et al., 2006), and the potential for tubing misconnections (Kimehi-Woods & Shultz, 2006). The IHI has published a number of perioperative FMEAs, including those for fire safety, risk of retained sponges, and wrong site surgery. The true value of an FMEA is that it can be conducted proactively, rather than reacting to published case reports of errors that have already occurred.

Descriptive studies

Descriptive studies have generated valuable evidence of the underlying causes of perioperative adverse events, such as anaphylaxis. French researchers (Mertes et al., 2004) evaluated 789 patients being referred for an anesthesia allergy consultation during a 2-year period for anaphylaxis or anaphylactoid reactions during anesthesia. The most frequent trigger of anaphylaxis was neuromuscular blocking agents (55%), the most common of which were succinyl-choline (37.6%) and Rocuronium (26.2%). The next most frequent triggering agents were latex (22.3%) and antibiotics (14.7%). These results were supported in a 6-year study in Norway, where neuromuscular blocking agents were found to trigger 93.5% of anaphylactic reactions (Harboe et al., 2005). These studies provide valuable evidence that anaphylaxis can occur in the operating room, and that perioperative nurses should be alert to this risk and ready to respond should an emergency occur.

Case reports

Case reports provide valuable evidence about the risk of serious, yet uncommon adverse events. These reports alert perioperative personnel of additional, sometimes unknown, risks, for which extra precautions or prevention should be directed. For example, a case report by Dauber and Roth (2009) describes a patient falling from an operating room bed used for spinal surgery. The authors conclude that the design of the bed makes it difficult to readily identify if it is in the locked position. The bed moved while transferring the patient from a gurney into the prone position. Being aware of this risk alerts healthcare providers to use extra caution when using this type of bed.

Another risk that is shared through case reports is surgical fires. When electrosurgery is used in the presence of an alcohol-based skin antiseptic, a fire can result. This risk has been highlighted many times, yet, surgical fires still occur as a result of this behavior (Batra & Gupta, 2008). Fires have also ignited when electrosurgery is used in the presence of oxygen built up under the surgical drapes. This risk has been highlighted in case reports, particularly in head and neck surgery and tracheostomy (Naftali et al., 2008; Niskanen et al., 2007; Weber et al., 2006). This knowledge alerts us to the importance of allowing flammable skin preparation agents to adequately dry and the vapors dissipate prior to applying the surgical drapes. It also heightens awareness of the importance of using the lowest concentration of oxygen necessary to maintain saturation, and tenting the drapes or otherwise exhausting the oxygen from under surgical drapes.

Other case reports alert us to the risk of using forced-air warming devices in a manner inconsistent with the manufacturer's recommendations. Forced-air warming devices are designed to distribute heat safely through a blanket, over a large surface area. When using the hose without the blanket, heat is not adequately distributed, and concentrates over smaller surface areas. Misusing forced-air warming devices without a blanket has resulted in second- and third-degree burns to patients (FDA, 2002).

Other sources of evidence

Expert opinion

When scientific evidence is not available to guide practice, perioperative nurses should seek expert opinion. This expertise is usually beyond the clinical expertise of individual practitioners or list serves. One way to identify experts is to seek out those who have published on the topic. This strategy can also be used to supplement evidence or to clarify points about the research. Professional associations may also be able to assist with identification of experts.

An example of this type of evidence in the operating room focuses on iodine allergies. Perioperative personnel are sometimes faced with the issue of a patient who is allergic to iodine or shellfish. Clinicians question the best alternative for skin antisepsis. The American Academy of Allergy Asthma and Immunology (2004) has addressed this issue in a position statement. IgE-mediated seafood allergy has never been attributed to iodine, but rather to specific proteins in fish and shellfish. Thus, fish or shellfish allergy does not indicate a sensitivity/allergy to iodine. And PVP–iodine skin antisepsis may be used for such patients.

Scientific principles

When research is not available to guide clinical decision making, scientific principles may be used to guide practice. For example, using the evidence about the half-life of prophylactic antibiotics provides guidance as to the best intraoperative redosing schedule. The half-life of cefazolin sodium is 1.8 h. Therefore, in surgeries lasting more than 2 h, redosing should be considered. This practice remains only partially implemented in perioperative settings. The knowledge gained through this scientific principle can be used to design perioperative practices to alert the anesthesia provider when redosing is recommended.

Manufacturers' instructions

Manufacturers' instructions are not scientific evidence. However, they do provide supportive rationale for how to safely use the high-tech equipment routinely found in the operating room. The design of medical devices is usually based upon scientific principles. For example, electrosurgical systems are designed by engineers with education and training in this field. The instructions are written to promote what these experts consider to be safe conditions. Misuse of electrosurgery has resulted in fires and patient burns.

Likewise, instructions for cleaning and sterilization of surgical instruments are also valuable information. Manufacturers often test the ability to adequately clean instruments and the parameters required to effectively sterile the item. Failure to follow these instructions can pose a serious infection control risk. Flexible endoscopes pose unique challenges for cleaning. Using the wrong valve has placed the patients at risk of transmission of HIV and hepatitis (Hepatitis, HIV cases confirmed at VA Hospital, 2009).

Clinical practice guidelines and perioperative standards

At times, the work of collecting and evaluating the evidence, and making recommendations for use, has been done through a clinical practice guideline. These guidelines incorporate the best available evidence, and often include consensus statements when addressing issues for which evidence is not as strong or missing. Some key clinical practice guidelines are listed in Table 6.2.

Practitioners should review these guidelines, evaluate their quality, and review more current evidence that might influence their adoptability.

National standards of practice provide excellent guidance as to the collective views of a nursing specialty. Perioperative standards developed by the Association of periOperative Registered Nurses provide guidance for a wide range of patient care issues, including such topics as cleaning, disinfection, and sterilization, use of a pneumatic tourniquet, electrosurgery, and lasers (AORN, 2009). These consensus documents incorporate the available published evidence. When this evidence is not available, the group uses collective expertise of committee members, consults with content experts,

Table 6.2 Selected perioperative clinical practice guidelines

Source	Guideline
American Academy of Orthopaedic Surgeons	Clinical guideline on prevention of symptomatic pulmonary embolism in patients undergoing total hip or knee arthroplasty
American College of Chest Physicians	Prevention of venous thromboembolism: American College of Chest Physicians Evidence-Based Clinical Practice Guidelines (8th edition)
American Society of Anesthesiologists	Practice guidelines for preoperative fasting and the use of pharmacologic agents to reduce the risk of pulmonary aspiration: application to healthy patients undergoing elective procedures
American Society of Anesthesiologists	Practice Guidelines for the Perioperative Management of Patients with Obstructive Sleep Apnoea
American Society of Health-System Pharmacists	ASHP therapeutic guidelines on antimicrobial prophylaxis in surgery
Centers for Disease Control and Prevention	Guideline for prevention of surgical site infection
National Collaborating Centre for Nursing and Supportive Care (NCC-NSC)	The management of inadvertent perioperative hypothermia in adults. (Commissioned by the National Institute for Health and Clinical Excellence (NICE). April 2008. http://www.rcn.org.uk/__data/assets/pdf_file/0006/197358/003_282.pdf
Royal College of Nursing (RCN)	Perioperative fasting in adults and children (full guideline). November 2005. RCN, London, UK. http://www.rcn.org.uk/__data/assets/pdf_file/0009/78678/002800.pdf

and uses scientific principles to make preliminary decisions. The draft document is posted on the web site www.aorn.org for public comment. Input is reviewed by the committee for consideration of inclusion. At times, this public comment results in additional evidence searches or consensus building to reach the final version of the document. Interested perioperative professionals are encouraged to participate in this public comment to assure that their voices are heard and that the documents reflect best practices.

Summary

The perioperative setting presents a unique context for patient care. The environment, equipment, and interventions are high tech and high risk. Therefore, the work of perioperative professionals is focused heavily on prevention of infection and injury. Perioperative patient care should be based upon the highest levels of evidence available to minimize the risk of infection and injury. However, focusing only on randomized clinical trials would exclude valuable knowledge that can and should be used to make clinical decisions. Practitioners should start with the highest levels of evidence (meta-analyses, randomized clinical trials), and systematically work down through non-experimental studies and lower the levels of evidence until they have arrived at the best clinical decision possible based upon available knowledge.

The context of the perioperative setting also poses unique challenges for the researcher. Much of what we know about perioperative patient safety has been gained from patient injuries reported in the literature. However, these injuries are seriously underreported, usually because of concern for negative perceptions and litigation. We do not know the true incidence or magnitude of these problems; retrospective study requires that a patient be injured in order for us to learn. Proactively studying processes through FMEA is currently underutilized, but may prove to be one of the most valuable methods for designing safe perioperative care in the future. This methodology can be used to develop interventions strategically focused on steps in processes that are at higher risk. The effectiveness of these interventions can then be evaluated using patient outcomes from large databases. In this way, we can move from a context of identifying risks to testing methods to minimize these risks.

The fast pace in the operating room and emphasis on efficiency of the surgery schedule also pose unique challenges. Critical thinking requires time, often away from patient care, and this must be part of a culture of inquiry to be accepted and supported by practitioners and leaders inside and outside of the operating room. This culture should be nurtured and integrated into all parts of the healthcare system in order to make the changes needed to provide optimum perioperative patient care.

Additional resources

AORN (2009). Recommended practices for prevention of unplanned hypothermia. In: *Perioperative Standards and Recommended Practices.* Denver, CO: AORN, Inc.

Mangram, A.J., Horan, T.C., Pearson, M.L., Silver, L.C., Jarvis, W.R. & the Hospital Infection Control Practices Advisory Committee (HIPAC). (1999). Guideline for prevention of surgical site infection. *Infection Control and Hospital Epidemiology*, 20, 250–278.

Pottinger, J.M., Starks, S.E. & Steelman, V.M. (2006). Skin preparation. *Perioperative Nursing Clinics*, 1, 203–210.

Stebral, L.L. & Steelman, V.M. (2006). Double gloving for surgical procedures: An evidence-based practice project. *Perioperative Nursing Clinics*, 1, 251–260.

Agency for Healthcare Research and Quality. www.ahrq.gov.

Association of periOperative Registered Nurses. www.aorn.org.

Cochrane Collaboration. www.cochrane.org.

Surgical Care Improvement Project (ND). www.medqic.org/dcs/ContentServ er?cid=1122904930422&pagename=Medqic%2FContent%2FParentSh ellTemplate&parentName=Topic&c=MQParents.

References

American Academy of Allergy Asthma and Immunology (2004). Academy position statement: The risk of severe allergic reactions from the use of potassium iodide for radiation emergencies. Available at http://www.aaaai.org/members/academy_statements/position_statements/potassium_iodide.asp (accessed August 17, 2009).

American Society of Anesthesiologists Task Force on Preoperative Fasting (1999). Practice guidelines for preoperative fasting and the use of pharmacologic agents to reduce the risk of pulmonary aspiration: Application to healthy patients undergoing elective procedures. *Anesthesiology*, 90, 896–905.

AORN (2009). Recommended practices for prevention of unplanned hypothermia. In: *Perioperative Standards and Recommended Practices.* Denver, CO: AORN, Inc.

Batra, S. & Gupta, R. (2008). Alcohol based surgical prep solution and the risk of fire in the operating room: A case report. *Patient Safety in Surgery*, 2, 10.

Borms, S.F., Engelen, S.L., Himpe, D.G., Suy, M.R. & Theunissen, W.J. (1994). Bair hugger forced-air warming maintains normothermia more effectively than thermo-lite insulation. *Journal of Clinical Anesthesia*, 6, 303–307.

Brady, M., Kinn, S. & Stuart, P. (2003). Preoperative fasting for adults to prevent perioperative complications. *Cochrane Database of Systematic Reviews*, Issue 4, Art. No.: CD004423. doi: 10.1002/14651858. CD004423

Dauber, M.H. & Roth, S. (2009). Operating table failure: Another hazard of spine surgery. *Anesthesia and Analgesia*, 108, 904–905.

DiazGranados, C.A., Jones, M.Y., Kongphet-Tran, T. et al. (2009). Outbreak of *Pseudomonas aeruginosa* infection associated with contamination of a flexible bronchoscope. *Infection Control and Hospital Epidemiology*, 30(6), 550–505.

Egorova, N.N., Moskowitz, A., Gelijins, A. et al. (2008). Managing the prevention of retained surgical instruments: What is the value of counting? *Annals of Surgery*, 247, 113–118.

Flores-Maldonado, A., Guzman-Llanez, Y., Castaneda-Zarate, S. et al. (1997). Risk factors for mild intraoperative hypothermia. *Archives of Medical Research*, 28, 587–590.

Flores-Maldonado, A., Medina-Escobedo, C.E., Ríos-Rodríguez, H.M. & Fernández-Domínguez, R. (2001). Mild perioperative hypothermia and the risk of wound infection. *Archives of Medical Research*, 32, 227–231.

Fossum, S., Hays, J. & Henson, M.M. (2001). A comparison study on the effects of prewarming patients in the outpatient surgery setting. *Journal of Perianesthesia Nursing*, 16, 187–194.

Frank, S.M., Beattie, C., Christopherson, R. et al. (1993). Unintentional hypothermia is associated with postoperative myocardial ischemia. The Perioperative Ischemia Randomised Anesthesia Trial Study Group. *Anesthesiology*, 78, 468–476.

Gawande, A.A., Studdert, D.M., Orav, E.J., Brennan, T.A. & Zinner, M.J. (2003). Risk factors for retained instruments and sponges after surgery. *New England Journal of Medicine*, 348, 229–235.

Germain, J.M., Carbonne, A., Thiers, V. et al. (2005). Patient-to-patient transmission of hepatitis C virus through the use of multidose vials during general anesthesia. *Infection Control and Hospital Epidemiology*, 26, 789–792.

Grossman, J. & Mackenzie, F.J. (2005). The randomized controlled trial: Gold standard, or merely standard? *Perspectives in Biology and Medicine*, 48(4), 516–534.

Guenaga, K.K.F.G., Matos, D. & Wille-Jørgensen, P. (2009). Mechanical bowel preparation for elective colorectal surgery. *Cochrane Database of Systematic Reviews*, Issue 1, Art. No.: CD001544. Available at http://mrw.interscience.wiley.com/cochrane/clsysrev/articles/CD001544/frame.html. doi: 10.1002/14651858.CD001544.pub3

Harboe, T., Guttormsen, A.B., Irgens, A., Dybendal, T. & Florvaag, E. (2005). Anaphylaxis during anesthesia in Norway: A 6-year single-center follow-up study. *Anesthesiology*, 102, 897–903.

Hepatitis, HIV cases confirmed at VA Hospital (2009). Infection control today. Available at http://www.infectioncontroltoday.com/hotnews/hepatitis-hiv-cases-va-hospital.html (accessed August 17, 2009).

Institute for Healthcare Improvement (ND). All FMEA tools. Available at http://www.ihi.org/ihi/workspace/tools/fmea/AllTools.aspx#16 (accessed August 17, 2009).

Kimehi-Woods, J. & Shultz, J.P. (2006). Using HFMEA to assess potential for patient harm from tubing misconnections. *Joint Commission Journal on Quality and Patient Safety*, 32, 373–381.

Kurz, A., Sessler, D.I. & Lenhardt, R. (1996). Perioperative normothermia to reduce the incidence of surgical-wound infection and shorten hospitalization. Study of Wound Infection and Temperature Group. *New England Journal of Medicine*, 334, 1209–1215.

Mangram, A.J., Horan, T.C., Pearson, M.L., Silver, L.C., Jarvis, W.R. & the Hospital Infection Control Practices Advisory Committee (HIPAC) (1999). Guideline for prevention of surgical site infection. *Infection Control and Hospital Epidemiology*, 20, 250–278.

Mason, D.S., Sapala, J.A., Wood, M.H. & Sapala, M.A. (1998). Influence of a forced air warming system on morbidly obese patients undergoing Roux-en-Y gastric bypass. *Obesity Surgery*, 8(4), 453–460.

Mertes, P.M., Laxenaire, M.C., Alla, F. & Groupe d'Etudes des Réactions Anaphylactoïdes Peranesthésiques (2004). [Anaphylactic and anaphylactoid reactions occurring during anesthesia in France. Seventh epidemiologic survey (January 2001–December 2002)]. *Annales Francaises d'anesthesie et de Reanimation*, 23(12), 1133–1143.

Murat, I., Berniere, J. & Constant, I. (1994). Evaluation of the efficacy of a forced-air warmer (Bair Hugger) during spinal surgery in children. *Journal of Clinical Anesthesia*, 6, 425–429.

Naftali, M., Jabaly-Habib, H. & Mukari, A. (2008). Burn during a routine pterygium excision operation. *European Journal of Ophthalmology*, 18, 639–640.

Ng, S.F., Oo, C.S., Loh, K.H., Lim, P.Y., Chan, Y.H. & Ong, B.S. (2003). A comparative study of three warming interventions to determine the most effective in maintaining perioperative normothermia. *Anesthesia and Analgesia*, 96, 171–176.

Niskanen, M., Purhonen, S., Koljonen, V., Ronkainen, A. & Hirvonen, E. (2007). Fatal inhalation injury caused by airway fire during tracheostomy. *Acta Anaesthesiologica Scandinavica*, 51(4), 509–513.

Pottinger, J.M., Starks, S.E. & Steelman, V.M. (2006). Skin preparation. *Perioperative Nursing Clinics*, 1, 203–210.

Royal College of Nursing (RCN) (2005). Perioperative fasting in adults and children (full guideline). London, UK: RCN. Available at http://www.rcn.org.uk/__data/assets/pdf_file/0009/78678/002800.pdf.

Stebral, L.L. & Steelman, V.M. (2006). Double gloving for surgical procedures: An evidence-based practice project. *Perioperative Nursing Clinics*, 1, 251–260.

Surgical Care Improvement Project (ND). Available at http://www.medqic.
org/dcs/ContentServer?cid=1122904930422&pagename=Medqic%2F
Content%2FParentShellTemplate&parentName=Topic&c=MQParents
(accessed August 17, 2009).

Tanner, J. & Parkinson, H. (2006). Double gloving to reduce surgical cross-
infection. *Cochrane Database of Systematic Reviews*, Issue 2, Art. No.:
CD003087. doi: 10.1002/14651858.CD003087.pub2

Thomas, S., Agarwal, M. & Mehta, G. (2001). Intraoperative glove perforation—single versus double gloving in protection against skin
contamination. *Postgraduate Medical Journal*, 77, 458–460.

US Food and Drug Administration (FDA) (2002). Burns from misuse of
forced-air warming devices. FDA Safety News: Show #9. Available at
http://www.accessdata.fda.gov/scripts/cdrh/cfdocs/psn/printer-full.
cfm?id=10 (accessed August 17, 2009).

U.S. HHS (2006). Eliminating serious, preventable, and costly medical errors—
never events. Centers for Medicare and Medicaid Services. Available at
http://www.cms.hhs.gov/apps/media/press/release.asp?Counter=1863
(accessed August 17, 2009).

Weber, S.M., Hargunani, C.A. & Wax, M.K. (2006). DuraPrep and the risk
of fire during tracheostomy. *Head and Neck*, 28, 649–652.

Wetterneck, T.B., Skibinski, K.A., Roberts, T.L. et al. (2006). Using failure mode and effects analysis to plan implementation of smart i.v. pump
technology. *American Journal of Health System Pharmacy*, 63(16),
1528–1538.

Wille-Jørgensen, P., Rasmussen, M.S., Andersen, B.R. & Borly, L. (2004).
Heparins and mechanical methods for thromboprophylaxis in colorectal
surgery. *Cochrane Database of Systematic Reviews*, Issue 1, Art. No.:
CD001217. doi: 10.1002/14651858.CD001217

Chapter 7

Midwifery in the context of new and developing technologies

Marlene Sinclair

Introduction

A major issue faced by midwifery at this time is the use of technology in childbirth. Birthing with or without technology is a contemporaneous issue that is complex, sensitive, and, for some clinicians, it is considered derisory. Creating technological solutions to human problems is an integral component of being human and we cannot halt the progress of innovation. As health professionals, information communication technology provides us with instant access to various forms of data including statistics, evidence-based guidelines, Cochrane reviews, etc. Electronic intelligent systems provide us with visible evidence about internal and external human functions. We live in a world where robotics is now employed in the management and delivery of pharmaceutical services, virtual training and e-learning are common practice. In vitro fertilization, intrauterine surgery, life support for 22-week-old babies, and over-the-counter abortificients are services routinely expected by the public and their expectations increase every day. The latest IT innovation is cloud computing technology, and very soon we will purchase handsets and browsers, log onto clouds for applications, widgets, etc., and we will not require software on our computers. Twitter, Facebook, MySpace, and BEBO are commonly used electronic social networks and more and more of us are logging on. Midwifery practice is changing too and women's birthing expectations are rapidly evolving to include expectations about diagnostic technologies to identify fetal abnormalities, sophisticated abortion techniques, painless childbirth using epidural technology, iphone applications for breast-feeding support, and online tutorials for labor and birth. The list is endless and the time is right for exploring in more depth what this is likely to mean for the context of midwifery in the future.

The aim of this chapter is to introduce the reader to contextual factors associated with midwifery practice within the context of the modern healthcare environment, which is technologically saturated with devices, techniques, and innovations. The physiological process of giving birth has not changed but what has changed is our rapid technological progress that is impacting on every aspect of midwifery, for example, mechanical devices (electronic fetal monitoring, EFM); education (e-learning); practice (tele-midwifery); bureaucracy (computerized maternity records); pharmacology (e-prescribing and epidural anesthesia). Every layer of the organization has been infiltrated by artificial intelligence systems that are insidious and invisible. Technology is at our disposal and midwives have major decisions to make with regard to using it appropriately for the health, safety, and well-being of mothers and babies.

Evidence of efficacy and effectiveness of technologies is a major challenge for all healthcare personnel. In the early phase of a technological innovation being adopted, it can be difficult to evaluate its effectiveness until relevant research is carried out. The life cycle of an item of healthcare technology comprises the stages of emergence, its introduction and adoption (in the clinical setting), and, if necessary, its modification and improvement—until finally it becomes obsolete and is replaced by a new model. Over this extended period, it is possible that misleading impressions of its benefits can hold sway, and Freemantle (1995), for example, would argue that only 20% of all healthcare technology has ever been formally evaluated. The use of EFM is an excellent example of this type of technology introduced without the necessary research and a Cochrane review by Alfirevic et al. (2006) concluded:

> There was no difference in the number of babies who died during or shortly after labour (about 1 in 300). Fits (neonatal seizures) in babies were rare (about 1 in 500 births), but they occurred significantly less often when continuous cardiotocograph (CTG)

was used to monitor fetal heart rate. There was no difference in the incidence of cerebral palsy, although other possible long-term effects have not been fully assessed and need further study. Continuous monitoring was associated with a significant increase in caesarean section and instrumental vaginal births. Both procedures are known to carry the risks associated with a surgical procedure although the specific adverse outcomes have not been assessed in the included studies.

However, in the UK, public and professional confidence has recently been raised as a result of the work of the Health Technology Assessment (HTA) program. The HTA is now part of the National Institute for Health Research (NIHR) and it is charged with producing independent research information about the effectiveness, costs, and broader impact of healthcare treatments and tests for those who plan, provide, or receive care in the NHS (http://www.hta.ac.uk/).

Defining healthcare technology

Technology in healthcare is still a relatively new concept and the UK Department of Health's Standing Committee on Technology (1992, p. 4) first defined healthcare technology as:

All the methods used by health professionals to promote health, to prevent and treat disease, and to improve rehabilitation and long term care. These methods include 'hardware' such as syringes, medicines and high technology diagnostic equipment; 'software' such as health education, diagnostic and therapeutic policies; as well as the skills and time of people working in the health services.

And its context to be:

The use of devices, equipment, drugs, procedures and care across the spectrum of medical, nursing and healthcare practice.

Defining birth technologies

These definitions are necessarily very broad but in my doctoral research (Sinclair, 1999) I classified the specific technologies (birth technologies) used in assisting childbirth.

"High" technology devices may or may not demand higher level of interpretative skill and expertise and I characterized these according to their electronically controlled automation and relative complexity in design or operation.

- High technology includes devices that are characterized by their electronically controlled automation—electronic intelligence.
- Low technology included mechanical devices such as the pinard stethoscope, which demand skill and expertise in interpretation and use by the midwife.

Further categorization included defining "Monitoring devices" such as the CTG machine and "Intervention Controlling" devices such as the IVAC® pump and the Graseby® infusion pump.

The devices such as the CTG machine, epidural syringe pump, dinomapp, and IVAC fit the hardware type of definition while midwives' usage of them fits the software dimensions, that is, the associated processes and skills.

It remains the case, of course, that interpretation arising from using such devices, of maternal or fetal condition, demands the skills and expertise of the midwife.

Understanding the complexity of technology and its relevance to midwifery

Martin Heidegger (1977, p. 297) stated: *technology comes to presence in the realm where revealing and unconcealment take place, where aletheia, truth, happens.* This is enlightening as it focuses my mind on the power of technology to show us what we do not routinely see and, in some instances, do not wish to see. In midwifery the power of technology to reveal what is not visible to the naked eye is evidenced in EFM in labor that provides us with an electronic graph of fetal well-being. Ultrasound can provide us with 3D pictures of fetuses and nuchal scanning can tell us whether or not a baby is likely to have Down syndrome. "Truth telling" is a core attribute. In 1983, Pacey drew attention to the human aspects of technology usage, organizational and cultural, that are difficult to reduce to identifiable principles and is known in the literature for his belief that our culture was fast moving toward thinking that technology could provide the appropriate "fix" whatever the problem.

In midwifery this is best observed in fetal medicine where it is now possible to save fetuses at 22 weeks gestation and use in vitro fertilization for artificial insemination. There are numerous examples but this one is an excellent demonstration of hope-filled human beings gaining their desired outcome as a direct result of technological progress and technological "fixing."

Philosophical perspectives on birth technology

Historically, science and technology have fondly been termed as bedfellows but there is substantive literary evidence in the past 50 years alone to indicate that philosophers are astute in their critical appraisal of technology. For example, in 1963, Ellul clearly identified that *technology produced values of unimpeachable merit, whilst simultaneously destroying values no less important* (p. 83) and it was therefore impossible to be sure about absolute progress or regress resulting from technological advances. After 25 years, Habermas (1987) identified that society now valued rationality and technical efficiency. Technology had become invisible in our society and Ihde (1990) was justified in interpreting our human value of technology as a form of evidence as it gave us power to view the human body as "hermeneutically transparent" and subject to analysis in the same way as a text. Soon the literature began to identify the problems and writers like Barnard (1997) drew attention to the loss of skill associated with clinicians becoming dependant on technology. He also identified the multilayered impact of technology on society and the administrative and bureaucratic infrastructure that was rapidly growing alongside innovative technologies.

Midwives and birth technology: major theoretical positions

In searching the literature for a demonstration of the views held by midwives about the phenomenon of birth technology, a diverse perspective emerges that echoes the comments made by Ellul over 50 years ago when he identified both negative and positive effects of technology, in general. The term "birth technology" is rarely mentioned in the literature prior to 1999. If we track some of the views we can see the Ellul's (1963) pattern emerging. For example, Wajcman (1991) held a very positive view of technology in childbirth and believed it was empowering and it gave women control over their childbirth experience. A very thought-provoking theory about good midwifery being the delicate balance between instinct, knowledge, and the judicious use of technology was posed by Hunt in 1992. In 1995, Dover and Gauge concluded that technology deskilled and disempowered the professional midwife. The following year midwives were accused of trusting the machines too much (Hemminki & Merilainen, 1996) and then several reports identify that technology is being used to control women (Barclay & Jones, 1996), denaturalizes childbirth (Cowie & Floyd, 1998), and gives power to the midwives (Purkiss, 1998). It was against this background of conflicting views that my doctoral research was undertaken to explore the perceived tensions between the so-called technocratic models of childbirth, where events and midwives' reactions may be largely guided by electronic and other devices, and the natural model in which midwives' role is to provide security and support for the mother as she births according to her own body's timetable (Sinclair, 1999). The study included 17 complete observations of induced birth defined as "technological," a survey of all practicing midwives in Northern Ireland at that time ($n = 1086$) and in-depth interviews with the midwifery managers ($n = 10$). Briefly summarized, the results showed that all midwives were comfortable with the use of technology in the labor ward, especially the use of the CTG and they rejected the possibility that they were overdependent on them. The technology was not considered to undermine the midwife's position, rather, it appeared to focus and strengthen it. Midwives reported problems experienced with technology and identified training needs. Women were positively disposed toward the use of technology and felt it enabled them to be on an equal par with the midwives and doctors. They valued the data from the CTG machine most of all and felt the evidence displayed on the screen and print out meant that nothing could be hidden from them. In the best instance of the use of the CTG machine, midwives were able to form a triangle and act as a conduit between the machinery, the women, and their partner.

Technology made everything transparent and I termed this concept as "revelatory." It included the power of the technology to reveal the inner world of their baby through the use of ultrasound and EFM. Factor analysis revealed that midwives did not trust machines too much and at that time midwives knew very little about evidence-based practice, guidelines, or electronic literature searching and they held very limited computing skills. Clinical observation demonstrated three types of midwives and two of these were previously identified in the literature (midwives who were depending on the technology and in danger of losing their skills and midwives who were using the technology to control the women). The new phenomenon to emerge was the midwife as conduit who was able to connect herself, the woman, and the machine to form a communicative, action-cycle or "triangle." In this situation, the midwife connected the processes of induction and the physiological changes taking place as labor progressed with evidence from the CTG machine and used the technology competently. In essence, the midwife had the confidence, intuition, and knows how to act as the conduit and normalize the event, therefore, using the technology appropriately as a support system.

The seminal work of Downe (2004), which is a major driving force for normal childbirth, has its origins in the Holocaust research undertaken by Antonovsky who theorized that individuals were able to deal with major life stressors when they felt a sense of coherence and belonging—what I term "connectedness." These characteristics are evident in supportive midwifery whether it is one-to-one care or team care. The confidence building and coping ability are interconnected and it is this support that the Cochrane review by Hodnett et al. (2007) refers to as being paramount in achieving optimal birth.

Birth technology competence

Crozier and colleagues (2006) produced seminal research exploring, analyzing, and confirming the role of the midwife in competent use of technology. Concept analyses, ethnographic fieldwork, and confirmatory focus groups were used to develop a theoretical model of midwifery competence in birth technology. Three midwife typologies were identified—"bureaucratic" where the guidelines and policy govern the midwives' decisions, "classical professional" where judgments are made based on personal expertise and experience, and "new professional" where women are involved in the decision making. The most common type was bureaucratic but it was possible for midwives to move from one typology to the other (Crozier et al., 2007).

Pregnant women's use of the Internet in pregnancy

Recent global research by Lagan et al. (2009) exploring pregnant women's use of the Internet across 25 countries demonstrated that both women ($n = 613$) and midwives ($n = 303$) were accessing the Internet. Midwives in Europe were referring more women to the Internet than those in North America and Oceania ($p = 0.01$), and midwives who were better educated were statistically more confident in advising women to read Internet-based information ($p = 0.036$).

The majority of pregnant women who completed the online questionnaire indicated they were accessing the Internet (97%) using common search engines to seek pregnancy-related information, social networking, support, and e-commerce. A large majority (94%) used the Internet to supplement information provided by health professionals and 83% of these used the information to make decisions about their pregnancy. Statistically, there was a significant increase in women's confidence levels with regard to making decisions about pregnancy following Internet searching ($p > 0.05$). Half of the women were dissatisfied with the information currently provided by health professionals.

Current context of midwifery care

Modern midwifery is practiced in a world in which knowledge transfer is becoming a global business that requires hardware, software, policy embedment, and appropriate finances to ensure its continued growth and success. Even though we have built electronic systems and pooled knowledge of clinical effectiveness and proposed NICE (National Institute for Health and Clinical Excellence) guidelines to impact on clinical practice, there is no guarantee that the care at the point of delivery in the woman's birthing journey through our health and social services is evidence informed. In our current systems of health, the old-fashioned ritualistic practices that offered a reasonable level of measurable care to every person within a confined unit have been ditched in favor of individualized care, also known as patient-centered, person-centered, and—from a midwifery perspective—women-centered care. With our sophisticated modern knowledge, we can design financial models for healthcare that are very sensitive to adjustments in terms of workforce data, capital changes, and mortality and morbidity statistics. However, it is important to find a balance between the goals of the institution, the government, the society, and the individual.

My recent clinical practice has been in a medium-sized maternity unit in Northern Ireland that facilitates birthing women with a choice between a homely, midwife-managed care package or a consultant-led obstetric package; here, the stark reality of competing demands for scarce staff was fully experienced. Regardless of expert managers, quality leadership, excellent physical resources, highly educated and motivated midwives, the balance between safe and unsafe care was always under threat. Unexpected emergencies in maternity care do happen and two or more lives are at stake—not one. Appropriate actions in obstetrical emergencies, such as cord prolapse, cardiac arrest, or pulmonary embolus, are difficult to prepare clinicians for, and paper-based evidence of mortality and morbidity is of little use to the clinicians on the ground. They need practice and the use of simulation exercises has been proven to be beneficial (Madden, 2008). The statistics, etiology, and recommended "effective" drug treatments are important, but evidence to do with practical management, effective support systems, and ensuring appropriate internalized knowledge in the minds and hands of those present is the type of knowledge required by the team, responsible for the delivery of effective care and management in an emergency situation. A summary of the main findings from recent clinical research on the management of obstetrical emergencies by Madden (2008) reported that "good teamwork depended on effective communication, multi-professional collaboration and control which could be adversely affected by inappropriate behaviours." The research recognized the important contribution of systems management, culture, social factors, environmental issues, multi-professional education, and reflection on practice through audit and research.

Evidence for midwifery practice needs to be contextually relevant, accessible, user-friendly, and effective. However, the application of knowledge is heavily dependent on individual action and the education and training of midwives is crucial. Education and training has changed substantially and evidence is part of the fabric that enshrines modern education. However, looking back over history to reflect on the enormity of change that has taken place since I began my midwifery practice in 1982 is a salutary reminder of the speed and direction of change. At that time, the bible for midwifery practice was a single publication by Margaret Myles (1981) titled *Textbook for Midwives* (9th edition). The first publication was in 1953 and currently we are reading the 15th edition by Fraser and Cooper, published in 2009. The difference between the editions is phenomenal and a factor of immense importance is noting that my 1981 edition did not have one reference and did not mention the word evidence or research. Reference to research first appeared in *The Midwives Rules*, in 1986 under the United Kingdom Central Council for Nursing, Midwifery and Health Visiting (UKCC) now the Nursing and Midwifery Council (NMC). Midwives were required to *demonstrate an awareness of research-based practice*. This was replaced by *able to use research in 1991 (UKCC)* and in the 2004 NMC *Midwives Rules practice should be based on the best available evidence*. Current midwifery textbooks are bursting with references and evidence-based guidelines and yearly updates or new editions are almost a necessity as new evidence is being produced everyday. The emerging problem is knowing how to manage knowledge translation, knowledge transfer, and knowledge dissemination. Recent publications focus on knowledge broker role and knowledge translation strategies and demonstrate the shift in our thinking about the need for and value of this type of evidence (Dobbins et al., 2009). However, some knowledge transfer is timeless and cultureless and midwives recognize that birthing is the business of women and, as an organic, physiological event, has not changed over time. The evidence required to support the naturalness of this phenomenon has been provided by NICE (2007) in their guidelines on intrapartum care when it was deemed necessary to state that "birth is not a medical event but a 'normal' process...and 90% of women will give birth to a single baby after 37 weeks with the baby presenting headfirst."

The influence of the midwife in promoting normal birth has been evidenced throughout history but now that we have access to modern electronic databases it is possible to gain a more truthful and balanced perspective of the individual and combined contribution made by midwives, men, physicians, philosophers, scientists, and women across the world, and over time, to childbirth. We can also *see* how birthing technologies have evolved from soft, mechanical, "low technologies" to the more "high technologies" with hardware diagnostic and artificially intelligent systems.

The midwifery model of care

The midwifery model of care, or social model of midwifery as it is sometimes referred to, has worldwide acceptance. It is based on a belief in physiological labor and the ability of a woman to birth without technological intervention such as epidural anesthesia, induction of labor, and EFM. The midwife is recognized as an expert in normal labor and birth and will refer women who need medical intervention to an obstetrician. Midwives are often referred to as "Guardians of normal birth." Normal birth was defined by the Royal College of Midwives in 2004:

> ... The majority of women with uncomplicated pregnancies are fit and healthy and have the potential to give birth normally with healthy newborns as the expected outcome. This is best met within a social model of care.
>
> Midwives are expert professionals skilled in supporting and maximizing normal birth and their skills need to be promoted and valued. The role of the midwife is integral to models of care, which promote normality ... The RCM recommends that midwives value, support and develop their own skills and knowledge and those of their colleagues, in the area of normal childbirth.

(RCM, 2004)

In the UK, data on the midwifery model of care/social model of midwifery is available on the BirthchoiceUK web site http://www. birthchoiceuk.com. This also contains data on UK home birth rates, which enable interesting comparisons to be made (see Table 7.1). The Royal College of Midwives' normal birth campaign web site http://www.rcm.org.uk/college/resources/campaign-for-normal-birth/ also contains useful data. This web site has excellent resource data on normal birth and of particular interest is a seminal work reviewing literature on pushing in labor. In the USA, information about

Table 7.1 UK home birth data from BirthchoiceUK database

Country	All birth (2007)	2007	2006	2005	2004	2003	2002	2001	2000	1999	1998
UK	765,317	2.68%	2.55%	2.41%	2.14%	2.06%	2.00%	1.90%	1.98%		
Northern Ireland	24,451	0.34%	0.39%	0.35%	0.38%	0.34%	0.21%	0.16%	0.24%		
Scotland	58,108	1.50%	1.36%	1.28%	1.12%	1.03%	1.01%	0.89%	0.94%	0.88%	0.87%
Wales	34,074	3.73%	3.53%	3.61%	3.06%	2.7%	2.15%	1.89%	2.23%	2.23%	2.14%
England	648,684	2.82%	2.69%	2.53%	2.25%	2.18%	2.15%	2.07%	2.13%	2.15%	2.2%

Source: From http://www.birthchoiceuk.com/BirthChoiceUKFrame.htm?http://www.birthchoiceuk.com/HomeBirthRates.htm.

the Midwives Model of Care can be found at http://cfmidwifery.org/ states/ and includes the following statement on the role of the midwife in maternity care provision:

- Monitoring the physical, psychological, and social well-being of the mother throughout the childbearing cycle.
- Providing the mother with individualized education, counseling, prenatal care, continuous hands-on assistance during labor and delivery, and postpartum support.
- Minimizing technological interventions.
- Identifying and referring women who require obstetrical attention.

Another example of support for the midwifery model can be found on an African web site http://www.blackmidwives.org/ offering pregnancy support, health promotion, and training. The organization is committed to empowering women, fathers, and families to have positive birth outcomes.

The UK's NICE guidelines on intrapartum care (NICE, 2007, http://www.nice.org.uk/nicemedia/pdf/CG55IPCQRGFINAL.pdf) emphasizes that "birth is not a medical event but a 'normal' process and as such clinical intervention should not be offered or advised where labor is progressing normally."

International definition of the midwife

The impact of internationalization on the profession is evidenced in the definition of "midwife" agreed by the International Confederation of Midwives (ICM), the World Health Organization (WHO), and the International Federation of Gynecology (FIGO) in 2005:

A midwife is a person who having been regularly admitted to a midwifery educational programme, duly recognized in the country in which it is located, has successfully completed the prescribed course of studies in midwifery and has acquired the requisite qualifications to be registered and/or legally licensed to practise midwifery.

The midwife is recognised as a responsible and accountable professional who works in partnership with women to give the necessary support, care and advice during pregnancy, labour and the postpartum period, to conduct births on the midwife's own responsibility and to provide care for the newborn and the infant. This care includes preventative measures, the promotion of normal birth, the detection of complications in mother and child, the accessing of medical care or other appropriate assistance and the carrying out of emergency measures.

The midwife has an important task in health counselling and education, not only for the woman, but also within the family and the community. This work should involve antenatal education and preparation for parenthood and may extend to women's health, sexual or reproductive health and childcare.

A midwife may practise in any setting including the home, community, hospitals, clinics or health units.

(International Confederation of Midwives, 2005)

This definition demonstrates the breadth and depth of the role of the midwife in caring for childbearing women and their families and the challenges for educationalists, researchers, and legislators to ensure the environment of care is conducive to maximizing the role of the midwife in the provision of effective and efficacious care. Midwives are committed to working in collaboration and partnership with public health agents in order to impact on global maternal and child health by ensuring adequate nutrition, clean water, and sanitation for all women in addition to the provision of competent midwifery services.

Global health: The World Health Organization

The WHO was established in 1951, and aimed to prevent the international spread of disease. Six "quarantinable" diseases: cholera, plague, relapsing fever, smallpox, typhus, and yellow fever were named. Global data were not available and modern telecommunications were in their infancy as most news traveled by telegram and boats were the major vehicle for travel. Today, world health is a major business supported by modern telecommunications technology, international data sets, and global policies. International conscience awareness of the health of the world population is now accepted and the achievement of the Millennium Development Goals (MDGs) is a shared goal for the world population.

Millennium development goals

In September 2000, 189 countries unanimously adopted the Millennium Declaration, pledging: "We will spare no effort to free our fellow men, women, and children from the abject and dehumanizing conditions of extreme poverty, to which more than a billion of them are currently subjected." The Declaration led to the articulation of eight MDGs, to be achieved between 1990 and 2015:

(1) eradicate Extreme Hunger and Poverty
(2) achieve Universal Primary Education
(3) promote Gender Equality and Empower Women
(4) reduce Child Mortality
(5) improve Maternal Health
(6) combat HIV/AIDS, Malaria, and other diseases
(7) ensure Environmental Sustainability
(8) develop a Global Partnership for Development.

Two of the eight MDGs concern maternal, newborn, and child health:

(1) Goal 4 is to reduce the mortality rate of children under the age of five.
(2) Goal 5 is to reduce the mortality rate of mothers and to achieve universal access to reproductive health.

The WHO launched the partnership for maternal, newborn, and child health in 2008 in an attempt to address the MDGs 4 and 5: "reducing child and maternal mortality and achieving universal access to reproductive health." This was a direct response to a rising concern over the health and social care profile of Asia and the Pacific: reported to have 41% of the 9.2 million children likely to die before they reached five in addition to 44% of the 500,000 pregnant women who die each year in childbirth and home to 55% of the world's women who would benefit from family planning services.

In May 2009, the WHO Assistant Director-General, Daisy Mafubelu, issued a statement to the world about the plight of mothers and the need for more midwives (regardless of gender) to save lives:

Every minute a woman dies during pregnancy or childbirth. This adds up to more than half a million women's lives lost every year with hardly any improvement since 1990. Most of these deaths occur in the developing world and most of these deaths are preventable.

> ...If we want to achieve Millennium Development Goal 5 and improve maternal health, we need to invest in midwives. Worldwide, more than 330 000 additional midwives are urgently needed. If based in a facility one midwife can attend up to 220 deliveries per year.

> ...WHO through its Department of Making Pregnancy Safer aims at strengthening the role of midwives and improving their education and training. Today, the Organization recognizes the contribution of midwives to the reduction of maternal and new-born mortality and renews its support to quality midwifery.

> (WHO, 2009)

Midwives are concerned and committed to the health and well-being of mothers, babies, fathers, and families. Therefore, in the context of modern midwifery practice, it is impossible for midwives of the world not to be concerned about the plight of women in countries where evidence demonstrates high rates of infant and maternal mortality are common, where there are no or few skilled birth attendants, inadequate transport, poor antenatal care, no maternity service provision, no sanitation, but an abundance of poverty and pain. WHO (2009) report 536,000 women die of complications during pregnancy and childbirth each year and the global maternal mortality rate is 400:100,000 but in Africa this figure is 900:100,000 (http://www.who.int/whosis/whostat/EN_WHS09_Part1.pdf) and the expenditure per capita on health in poor countries is US$ 16, compared to US$ 2672 in high-income countries (WHO, UNICEF, UNFPA and World Bank, 2007). Living in an affluent society, like that of the UK, can be a challenge when a midwife has experienced maternity services in one of the poorer countries. Excellent midwifery services are available in the UK and this was evidenced in the Healthcare Commission Report (2007).

> ... Overall, the vast majority of women reported a positive experience of the care received during pregnancy and during their labour and the birth with nine in ten rating the care they received as "excellent", "very good" or "good". More than three quarters of respondents reported that they had always been spoken to in a way they could understand, treated with respect and dignity, and treated with kindness and understanding at these stages of care.

Without the Internet we would not have instant access to recent data on world health statistics, and it is important for the future of health and social care to ensure that as many countries as possible have access to the Internet and work in partnership to achieve the millennium goals.

Global statistics on Internet usage

Statistics on World Internet Users and Population Stats for 2009 provides clear evidence of the major developments that have taken place globally in international communications over the past 10 years. More than one billion people surf the Internet every month and developing countries are getting more connected. For example, data for Africa indicate 65,903,900 Internet users but this accounts for only 6.7% population penetration. However, since 2000 this is the country with the highest growth, presenting a 1359.9% increase. In Europe we see a record of 402,380,474 users with a 50.1% population penetration and a growth rate of 282.95%. In Australia there is a record of 20,838,019 users, and a population penetration of 60.1% with a growth rate of 173.4%. However, Asia is reported to have the highest Internet usage with 389 million surfers each month and Asia is home to 35.6% of all Internet surfers. In North America 70 out of 100 people surf the net, 53:100 in Australia. Factually, more than one billion people surf the Internet each month. The evidence of international connectivity is overwhelming and the majority of midwives can connect to the global information highway to communicate at social, professional, and academic levels with midwives, health professionals, and women, instantaneously.

Inappropriate use of technology

In 1985, the WHO held a consensus conference in Brazil on the appropriate use of technology in childbirth. Induction technology had become so sophisticated and there was concern of its overuse and abuse. Twenty-one recommendations were made and one of these was the recommendation that "birth should not be induced for convenience, and induction should not take place unless there was a medical reason." However, the inappropriate use of technology continues (Sinclair & Gardner, 2001; Wagner, 1994) and although its creation was to reduce maternal and infant morbidity and mortality, the very act of interference with a normal physiological way of birthing leads to a complex chain of events we named the "technological cycle" and includes strict antenatal monitoring, active management of labor, an increased use of induction of labor, continuous EFM, epidural analgesia, episiotomy, birthing in the lithotomy position, and increased risk of instrumental birth (Hatamleh et al., 2008; Sinclair, 1999; Sinclair & Crozier, 2004).

Use of technology during pregnancy and childbirth

Research by Hatamleh et al. (2008) reported on a convenience sample of 200 primigravidae women giving birth in Jordan and mapped their exposure to and acceptance of technology in childbirth. The results are challenging. First of all active management led to no maternal deaths, no uterine rupture, and no cord prolapse. However, five infants died at birth, all were twins and the cause of death in each was registered as respiratory distress syndrome due to prematurity. The majority of births were supported, managed, and controlled by the use of technology. The more the women were exposed to technology the better they perceived their care. Ultrasound scanning ranged from 1 to 27 (mean 9.7, SD = 5.4) and the majority of women expected to be scanned at every visit. Qualitative data demonstrated that women perceived the quality of their care to be better if they had more scans and more EFM in the antenatal and intranatal setting. Women reported a need to "see" how well their baby was growing. Induction was the "norm" with 161/200 (80.5%) being induced. A range of technological interventions was recorded: 144 (72%) women had an artificial rupture of membranes, 145 (72.5%) had their labor augmented with oxytocin, 178 (89%) had continuous EFM, and 132 (66%) had an episiotomy. Half of the babies ($n = 100$, 50%) were admitted to the neonatal care unit for resuscitation; their length of stay in the neonatal unit ranged from 1 h to 18 days. Prophylactic antibiotics were administered to all women as part of the care package. In the postnatal period, many women reported feeling pain at the episiotomy site on the tenth day ($n = 83$, 42%), painful intercourse at 6 weeks ($n = 81$, 41%), high temperature with shivering ($n = 54$, 27%), infection at the episiotomy site ($n = 28$, 14%), mastitis ($n = 24$, 12%), urinary incontinence ($n = 19$, 9.5%), and fecal incontinence ($n = 4$, 2.5%). Subsequent regression analyses of the data demonstrated that the technological cycle of induction was in operation and confirmed the potential for morbidity. Indeed this is a complex picture but it needs to be considered carefully as it was a convenience sample, there were no comparative data and the overall statistical profile on paper would support active management of labor. In essence, we have an excellent example of technology producing both beneficial and not so beneficial outcomes. The challenge remains—to use it effectively and efficaciously.

Conclusion: the Instantaneous Age and the role of modern technology in childbirth

With commitment to listening to what women want and the agenda for choice, it is important for midwives to be aware of the fact that there is evidence to prove that women given choices will choose induction and cesarean section over the natural childbirth experience. A large Illinois study of 2.3 million women over a 12-year period reported 25–30% of women are choosing to have their labor timed and started as opposed to starting spontaneously (Murthy et al., 2004).

We are currently living in the Instantaneous Age in which the barriers of distance and transport have been drastically reduced with the use of computers and satellite technology. For the ancient practice of organic midwifery it is no surprise to find tension between the technocratic and natural models of childbirth. The technocratic model—where events and midwives' reactions may be largely guided by electronic and other devices—and the natural model in which the midwives' role is to provide security and support for the mother as she births according to her own body's timetable.

Modern midwifery takes place in an electronically connected web of seamless and endless activity in which distance is dissolved by access to the Internet. The world is indeed a smaller place in which we no longer rely on birds, horses, or telegrams to communicate effectively, and the health professional is no longer the gatekeeper to a hidden body of knowledge. Evidence for practice can be retrieved from the Internet within seconds. Health professionals and pregnant women and their partners have access to the same information available on the Internet and this is indeed a challenge for the future preparation of health and social care practitioners. New professionals need to develop critical appraisal skills and be confident working in partnership with women to seek, appraise, and act on valid and reliable evidence freely accessible from the Internet. Midwives need to embrace technologies "high" and "low," "hard" and "soft" with conviction and professional confidence in the ability to use them wisely and judiciously for the betterment of the health and well-being of mothers and babies across the world.

References

Alfirevic, Z., Devane, D. & Gyte, G.M.L. (2006). Continuous cardiotocography (CTG) as a form of electronic fetal monitoring (EFM) for fetal assessment during labour. *Cochrane Database of Systematic Reviews*, Issue 3, Art. No.: CD006066. Available at http://www.cochrane.org/reviews/en/ab006066.html. doi: 10.1002/14651858.CD006066

Barclay, L. and Jones, L. (1996). *Midwifery: Trends and Practice in Australia*. Australia: Churchill Livingstone.

Barnard, A. (1997). A critical review of the belief that technology is a neutral object and nurses are its master. *Journal of Advanced Nursing*, 26, 126–131.

Cowie, J.L. & Floyd, S.R. (1998). The art of midwifery: Lost to technology? *Australian College of Midwives Incorporated Journal*, 11(3), 20–24.

Crozier, K., Sinclair, M., Kernohan, W.G. & Porter, S. (2006). Birth technology competence: A concept analysis. *Evidence Based Midwifery*, 43(3), 96–100.

Crozier, K., Sinclair, M.K., Kernohan, W.G. & Porter, S. (2007). The development of a theoretical model of midwifery competence in birth technology. *Evidence Based Midwifery*, 5(4), 119–124.

Department of Health. (1992). *Assessing the Effects of Health Technologies: Principles, Practice, Proposals*. London: Department of Health.

Dobbins, M., Robeson, P., Clliska, D. et al. (2009). A description of a knowledge broker role implemented as part of a randomized trial evaluating three knowledge translation strategies. *Implementation Science*, 4, 23. doi 10.1186/1748-5908-4-23

Dover, S.L. & Gauge, S.M. (1995). Fetal monitoring—midwifery attitudes. *Midwifery*, 11(1), 18–27.

Downe, S. (2004). *Normal Childbirth Evidence and Debate*. Edinburgh: Churchill Livingstone.

Ellul, J. (1963). The technological order. In: Mitcham, C. & Mackey, R. (eds) *Philosophy and Technology*. New York: The Free Press, pp. 86–105.

Fraser, D. & Cooper, A. (2009). *Myles Textbook for Midwives*, 15th ed. Edinburgh: Churchill Livingstone, Elsevier.

Freemantle, N. (1995). Dealing with uncertainty: Will science solve the problems of resource allocation in the UK NHS? *Social Science and Medicine*, 40(10), 1365–1370.

Gelbart, N.R. (1998). *The King's Midwife: A History and Mystery of Madame Du Coudray*. Berkeley and Los Angeles: University of California Press.

Hatamleh, R., Sinclair, M., Kernohan, W.G. & Bunting, B. (2008). Technological childbirth in northern Jordan: Descriptive findings from a prospective cohort study. *Evidence Based Midwifery*, 6(4), 130–135.

Habermas, J. (1987). *The Theory of Communicative Action: A Critique of Functionalist Reason* (T. McCarthy, Trans. Vol. 2 Lifeworld and System). London: Polity Press.

Healthcare Commission (2007) Women's experiences of maternity care in the NHS in England. Available at http://www.cqc.org.uk/_db/_documents/Maternity_services_survey_report.pdf.

Heidegger, M. (1977). The question concerning technology. In: Krell, D.F. (ed.) *Basic Writings*. New York: Harper & Row (original work published in 1954), pp. 287–317.

Hemminki, E. & Merilainen, J. (1996). Long term effects of caesarean sections: Ectopic pregnancies and placental problems. *American Journal of Obstetrics and Gynecology*, 174(5), 1569–1574.

Hodnett, E.D., Gates, S., Hofmeyr, G.J. & Sakala, C. (2007). Continuous support for women during childbirth. *Cochrane Database of Systematic Reviews*, Issue 2, Art. No.: CD003766. doi: 10.1002/14651858. CD003766.pub2

Hunt, S. (1992). A matter of feelings. In: Jowit, M. & Kargar, I. (eds) *Radical Midwifery Celebrating 21 Years of ARM*. Ormskirk: Association of Radical Midwives.

Ihde, D. (1990). *Technology and the Lifeworld: From Garden to Earth*. Bloomington: Indiana University Press.

International Confederation of Midwives. (2005). *Definition of the Midwife*. The Hague: ICM.

Lagan, B.M., Sinclair, M., Kernohan, W.G. (2009). A web-based survey of midwives' perceptions of women using the Internet in pregnancy: A global phenomenon. *Midwifery*, doi:10.1016/j.midw.2009.07.002. Available online August 22, 2009.

Madden, E. (2008). Inter-professional collaboration in obstetric emergencies. Unpublished PhD Thesis, University of Ulster, UK.

Murthy, K., Grobman, W.A., Lee, T.A. & Holl, J.L. (2004). Racial disparities in term induction of labor rates in Illinois. *Medical Care*, 46(9), 900–904.

Myles, M. (1981). *Textbook for Midwives*, 9th ed. Edinburgh: Churchill Livingstone.

National Institute for Clinical Excellence (NICE) (2007). Available at http://www.nice.org.uk/nicemedia/pdf/CG55IPCQRGFINAL.pdf.

Nursing and Midwifery Council (NMC) (2004). *Midwives Rules and Standards*. London: NMC.

Pacey, A. (1983). *The Culture of Technology*. Oxford: Blackwell.

Purkiss, J. (1998). The medicalisation of childbirth. *MIDIRS Midwifery Digest*, 8(1), 110–112.

Royal College of Midwives (RCM) (2004). Available at http://www.rcm. org.uk/college/standards-and-practice/position-statements/.

Sinclair, M.K. (1999). Midwives' readiness to use high technology in the labour ward. Implications for education and training. Unpublished PhD Thesis, Queen's University, Belfast.

Sinclair, M.K. & Gardner, J. (2001). Midwives' perceptions of the use of technology in assisting childbirth in Northern Ireland. *Journal of Advanced Nursing*, 36(2), 229–236.

Sinclair, M. & Crozier, K. (2004). Medical device raining in maternity care: Part 2. *British Journal of Midwifery*, 12(8), 509–513.

United Kingdom Central Council (UKCC) (1986). *Midwives Rules*. London: UKCC.

United Kingdom Central Council (UKCC) for Nursing Midwifery and Health Visiting (1991). *A Midwife's Code of Practice*. London: UKCC.

Wagner, M. (1994). *Pursuing the Birth Machine*. London: Ace Graphics.

Wajcman, J. (1991). *Feminism Confronts Technology*. Oxford: Polity Press.

World Health Organization (1985). Appropriate technology for birth. *Lancet*, 11(8452), 436–437.

World Health Organization (2009). Midwives: A worldwide commitment to women and the newborn—statement of Daisy Mafubelu. Available at http://www.who.int/making_pregnancy_safer/events/news/international_ day_midwife/en/print.html.

WHO, UNICEF, UNFPA & World Bank (2007), *Maternal Mortality in 2005: Estimates Developed by WHO, UNICEF, UNFPA and the World Bank*. Geneva: WHO.

Chapter 8

Making context work in mental health

Dawn Freshwater and Jane Cahill

Introduction

Mental health care, as with other health-related disciplines, has been pressured to perform in terms of research and evidence-based practice. In addition, global reform has led to governments of Westernized countries producing national guidelines based upon the best available evidence for the best treatment of various mental health conditions (Freshwater & Stickley, 2007). In this chapter we focus on the context of evidence as developed and applied in mental health care settings. In particular, we employ two examples of how evidence can be used to both define and influence practice environments and subsequently impact care; these being the process of benchmarking and the practice of reviewing research and research evidence. Our narrative draws upon contemporary and international research studies in the mental health field, and, where appropriate, current policies, procedures, and evidence-based guidelines are incorporated to underpin the discussion.

We begin with a brief overview of mental health care and the context of its development. Subsequently, we describe and discuss the ways in which benchmarking and peer-review processes both subtly and more overtly inform clinical practice and patient care. Finally we bring the focus back to patient care and research that seeks to understand the patient's experience.

Contextualizing mental health care

The postwar history of global health care systems has seen the closing down of large mental institutions such as asylums, or places of safety, as they were known. From 1880 to 1950, specifically in Europe, but in many Westernized countries, the asylum was the chief source of care for the mad, the lunatic, and the insane. However, as Freshwater (2003) notes, thousands of people with mental illness that were cared for in these vast institutions were out of sight and out of mind and places that were meant to be places of safety in many cases became places of neglect. Some of these old hospitals certainly did become grim places and this, coupled with a growing humanitarian view that the mentally ill were scandalously treated, led to a belief that the walls of the old institutions should be pulled down and the inmates released into the outside world. Academics and radical academia played its part in this debate; attacks rained down on authoritarian psychiatry and the culture of hard drugs and electroconvulsive therapy. The closure of the institutions meant that mental health care was substituted by care in the community. The idea being that resources tied up in the buildings and their beds would be released to provide a support service for the mentally ill once they were returned to their families and communities. The reality, however, was and continues to be rather more problematic than at first envisaged.

The problem of how to manage the mental health of the population is a very real one. By 2020 the World Health Organization (WHO) warns that deaths from mental health disorders will be the second most common cause of morbidity. Fewer than 40% of primary care–focussed professionals, such as GPs, have any postgraduate training in psychiatry (Ward, 2008), with less than 2% of nurses in generic primary care having any training in mental health care (Crosland & Kai, 1998). Whilst some of these figures were reported nearly a decade ago, little has changed since then (Freshwater, 2007).

Whilst there are many new imperatives to address these concerns, high-quality evidence-based mental health care in the community is doomed to fail if it is not given the attention it both deserves and demands. Care in the community is, essentially, a good idea. It is known that the damage done to patients by incarceration is directly proportional to the length of time spent in an institution.

The question, though, is not about if there should be mental health provision in primary care, but rather what type of community care is needed. Answering this question involves speaking to people, to carers, to users, listening to their narratives, and taking them seriously.

Sadly research, policy, and practice in mental health care not only emphasize short-term care, which is not surprising given the "toxic speed sickness" that we currently suffer from, but also focus on the issue of compulsion, the use of legal powers to commit patients to hospital against their will. These take priority over understanding the underlying causes that lead to a mental health crisis in the first place. What we would call *scare* in the community has moved us into a phase of moral panic based on received wisdom not constructed knowledge (Belenky et al., 1986). As authors, this raises questions about the way in which we can support the development of constructed knowledge within mental health context. Critical review of processes and understanding of how evidence is generated and knowledge is constructed within this context is desperately needed and it is to this that we attend in the remainder of this chapter.

The available facts and figures (e.g., the WHO web site, http://www.who.int/mental_health/en/) give an indication of the increased prevalence of mental illness in contemporary society. But what is the cause of this increase. Furthermore has there really been an increase in mental illness? We have to consider that we now have labels and diagnoses that enable previously undiagnosed symptoms and behaviors to be identified, categorized, and reported. There has been a long-held belief that patients' symptoms of mental distress can be categorized (*The Diagnostic and Statistical Manual of Mental Disorders* [DSM] is used by the American Psychiatric Association [APA] to classify mental disorders). This has been widely contested. But perhaps now there is less stigma around mental illness and maybe more people feel able to report their symptoms and, of course, record-keeping mechanisms have now become more efficient. These factors may all contribute to the increasing figures. But what are the contextual factors that influence our mental health and indeed create the mental illness of the future? The development of a body of knowledge around mental health will help to elucidate these issues; however, the nature of the evidence and knowledge generated also needs to be fully addressed.

The practice of reviewing: the evolution of scientific literature

Whilst evidence-based practice has become the cornerstone of contemporary health care, the question of what constitutes evidence is still open to debate. The hierarchy of evidence model in which randomized controlled trials (RCTs) are explicitly prized not only determines what best evidence is, but also the degree to which research that is clinically focussed and practice driven can carry equal weight in its influence on practice and practitioners. As you will by now have grasped, the hierarchy of evidence model explicitly determines how research is rated both in regard to funding and success of grant applications and quality of research outputs, which can include research papers, book chapters, and research reports. In this sense it also determines the focus of much mental health research. Research is often invoked as a method of establishing whether or not to provide a service, or which service to provide (Parry, 1996, p. 282). However, the huge amount of research conducted into areas such as psychological therapy over the last 40 years, has to a large extent failed to influence the design of either services or treatments. Parry (1996, p. 286) argues that "it is hard to point to an example of major changes in service delivery attributable to research." Where research has demonstrated that a particular type of treatment would benefit patients, service providers have not always ensured that the skill base is developed. One such example of this is the strong evidence that the therapeutic relationship is the sine qua non of successful therapy. And yet the present focus is on effectiveness of short-term interventions such as cognitive-behavioral and psychosocial skills, which are of course important but where often, although not always, the relationship comes second best to outcome when actually the relationship is the outcome.

In many countries judgments of the quality of research are measured and made across three main categories; these being research outputs, research environment, and research esteem (e.g., the UK Research Assessment Exercise [RAE], now the Research Excellence Framework [REF], is similar to initiatives in Australia and New Zealand and the USA). Publication of papers in peer-reviewed journals has long been regarded as an international indicator of both the quality and the significance of research in professional areas, and as such provides evidence of research outputs and is an indicator of research esteem. Bishop (2004) notes that dissemination is a vital link between research, development, and changing practice. However, it is also crucial that new knowledge is made accessible to practitioners, who can use such knowledge to improve care delivery needs, and managers, who have the ability to facilitate change in policy and practice. Health care research and evidence for best practice then must relate in some way to service delivery, professional development, and/or knowledge generation.

Whether you are an undergraduate student of health care practices, or already a qualified practitioner working clinically in education or/and in research, reading and critiquing journal papers will be something that you are familiar with and indeed it will be woven into the very fabric of your professional development. In international research assessment exercises, published papers are assessed on their originality, significance, and rigor as demonstrated by "the extent to which knowledge, theory or understanding in the field has been increased or practice has been (or is likely to be) improved" (Freshwater, 2007). Using standardized pointers such as impact factor, immediacy index, and cited half-life, the Institute for Scientific Information provides databases which in turn can offer useful insights into the communication of scholarly research. For further, detailed information follow the link http://admin-apps.isiknowledge.com/JCR/JCR?SID=W1%40 lkJOh8dnHjgK4Ef8 for Web of Knowledge Journal Citation reports, where one can access definitions and explanations regarding the nature of impact factor, immediacy impact, and cited half-life.

However, as Amin and Mabe (2000, p. 6) remind us, these factors are not the only measures and are not altogether reliable, affected by "subject area, type, and size of journal and the 'window of measurement' used." Many journals and indeed practitioners debate and question the value of the impact factor and how easily it can be influenced by such practices as self-citation and plagiarism through redundant and duplicate publications and problematic editorial practices.

In the context of this chapter, we might ponder:

- What makes a scholarly paper?
- How does the generation of evidence link to the publication of research?
- How does evidence published in journals inform and transform practice?
- How does the process of peer review contribute to and influence practice environments?

The answers to these questions are of course multifaceted and open to debate. For this chapter we particularly wish to highlight the context of evidence and knowledge production in mental health care through examination of the peer-review process. Given that this chapter is focussing on the evidence base for mental health practice, we will be using data to support our claims regarding the peer-review process drawn from an international impact-factored mental health journal. Peer review essentially acts as a quality control mechanism, maintaining standard of efficacy, ethics, and validity of what goes into print and in turn what does and does not influence practice. Quality control is a well-known process that underpins evidence-based paradigms, but its presence in the peer-review process is not always transparent. The audit trail for the peer-review process is not always evident and there is little or no obvious symmetry with the rigor of the methodology underpinning the hierarchy of evidence model. Freshwater (2005, p. 387) challenges readers, authors, and researchers alike to "interrogate the fundamental assumptions upon which the peer review is based."

In essence practitioners, researchers, and educators place a lot of faith in the peer-review process with little critical appraisal of the context in which it takes place. We would argue that reviewers and the peer-review process politicizes knowledge production and in this regard is a contextual factor for all practitioners appraising and implementing evidence in mental health care settings. Knowledge generated from the peer-review process can be heavily loaded and is sometimes derived from flimsy evidence. Notwithstanding our misgivings concerning the peer-review process, if viewed in this context, that is of a story that perpetuates other stories, it is of course a helpful tool, if used responsibly and rigorously, to understand the stories that inform practice and health care discourse in general. With this caveat we now wish to turn our attention to the specifics of reviewing practice—in this case a review of peer-reviewed material relating to psychiatric and mental health practice conducted by the authors of this chapter.

Over the past three decades there have been a number of reviews of psychiatric and mental health literature. Davis (1981) in a review of articles published between 1971 and 1980 observed that a significant number of articles focussed on the role of the practitioner, a finding echoed by O'Toole (1981) who found that 30% of the studies were too focussed on the role of the practitioner. Jones and Jones (1987) noted a trend for research to increase in scientific rigor over time and to write better in terms of clarity and sophistication of research design. The two most recent reviews concentrated on treatment outcomes (Merwin & Mauck, 1995), and issues of study quality (Yonge et al., 1997).

The authors of this chapter, both with considerable mental health expertise, undertook a study that was essentially a systematic review of peer-reviewed research articles. In regard to systematic reviews and meta-analytic studies, a more robust and expansive explanation of the construction of both can be accessed via the web site http://www.york.ac.uk/inst/crd/SysRev/!SSL!/WebHelp/SysRev3.htm.

These articles were published in one impact-factored journal—*The International of Journal of Psychiatric and Mental Health Nursing* (of which the first author is editor)—with the aim of providing not only a contemporary comment on the evidence being generated for best practice in mental health settings, but, and more importantly, on how mental health care is influenced by the context of dominant research discourses upheld by peer-review processes in the mental health literature. Review methodology itself is premised on the concept of an inextricable link and dependant relationship between research and practice: research assists in provision of scientific basis for mental health care, provides support for allocation of resources, and identifies areas of good practice and recommendations for further research. Hence research "furnishes an increased understanding of practice and assists nurses in modifying their activities to provide the best nursing care possible, *if research and practice are linked*" (emphasis added) (Yonge et al., 1997).

The review, which we cite as an example, was also explicitly premised on a relationship between research and practice, but we acknowledge that applying research findings in health care practice is perhaps one of the biggest challenges facing the allied health professions. A number of barriers to the effective integration of research and practice have been identified—these include access, attitude, institutional support, and occupational culture. The review was undertaken accessing journal papers over a 6-year time span (2003–2008 inclusive). The entire population of published studies was covered in the JPMHN over the 6-year time span (rather than selecting a sample of studies). Several questions were formulated in order to understand the data available and to make sense of the relationship between research and practice:

- What kinds of research are being conducted?
- What are the dominant measures and methodologies?

- What are the sample and setting characteristics of the research?
- What are the key content areas?
- How is nursing practice and nursing profession formulated and configured?

Interpreting the evidence

Type of research

The results indicate that over the 2003–2008 time span, the majority (65%) of articles were based on primary research with 21% based on secondary research (derived from preexisting datasets). A small proportion of studies concerned measure development and validation studies (5%). The dominant methodological approach *within* primary research appeared to be qualitative: of the 361 studies 217 (60%) were qualitative. This trend was basically stable over the time span although a decrease was observed in 2008 with 30/68 (44%) primary research articles based on qualitative methods. A range of evaluation activity including controlled and uncontrolled trial designs, cohort, longitudinal and prospective studies, and case studies was also well represented (75/361: 21%) along with surveys (19%). Within the secondary research studies, the majority were nonsystematic literature reviews (93%): this pattern was largely consistent across the time span.

Content focus of articles

The results indicate that in JPMHN, clinical issues (62%) and issues relating to nursing practice (68%) dominate as topic areas over the 6-year time period. Year on year the proportion of studies examining clinical issues remains over 50% and for nursing practice, proportions examining this issue peak from 2004 to 2006 with almost three quarters of articles focussing on this issue. Within the category "nursing practice," the most common topic tended to be issues relating to aspects of professional practice. These covered attitudes, knowledge, role, training, outcome assessment, research and practice, clinical supervision, and therapeutic relationships. Over the time period this proportion peaked in 2005 at 41%. Social issues did not tend to be a common topic area, although there are indications that over the 6 years there were modest increases in the proportions of these articles being published.

Characteristics of samples

JPMHN published predominantly articles using either patient service/user samples (46%) or nurse/health practitioner samples (46%). Over the time period the proportion of studies based on nurse/health practitioner samples peaked in 2005 at 61% before returning to 2003 levels, while studies using patients/service users correspondingly decreased in 2005 (38%) before increasing to 45% by 2008. Other population groups that were represented included carers (5%), families (4%), and students and women (3%).

Setting characteristics

The results show that research was conducted in or related to predominantly acute inpatient (24%) or community mental health settings (19%). For the latter, there was a marked increase subsequent to 2003. Education (i.e., institutions offering nursing courses) and forensic settings were also represented, each accounting for approximately 5% articles over the time period. Articles reporting research based around forensic settings showed a marked decline from 2003.

Measures

In the JPMHN studies, the 93 measures were used a total of 107 times. In terms of the focus of these measures, 68 (73%) focussed on clients, 16 (17%) focussed on practitioners, 2 (2%) focussed on caregivers, 3 (3%) focussed on families, and 4 (4%) focussed on the work environment. Of the 68 client-focussed measures, 29% pertained to psychiatric symptoms and psychological distress, 18% to risk assessment/management issues, 12% to psychosis/severe mental health, 12% to emotional problems/well-being issues, 4% to interpersonal problems, 9% to functioning/quality of life issues, 7% to health/needs assessment, and 1% to eating disorders and substance abuse. Of the 16 practitioner-focussed measures, the majority were related to attitudes toward risk (7: 44%) and staff stress/burnout (7: 44%). Eight (9%) of the 93 studies used new measures that were presented for the first time in the study. The results indicate that a client perspective was used in 50% of measures and a practitioner perspective in 46% measures. For a small proportion of measures (5%), caregivers'/family members' perspectives were used.

Implications of "context" for practice: effect of peer review on practice

The effect of context—that is the context of peer-review process and the review of peer-reviewed material—on mental health practice is complex and multilayered. The peer-review process in itself is a powerful and authoritative voice which lends weight to the power imbalance in the practitioner–patient relationship. We would argue that it privileges some mental health treatments over others, and has implications for future research activity and subsequently treatments for further investment. It follows then that, as a result of published research, access to some less well-established treatments will be limited. From the perspective of the practitioner and researcher, certain theoretical models will be supported/highlighted with other more creative, contentious, or polemic models marginalized and isolated. Furthermore the language used to communicate evidence for best practice may further isolate carers and users of those services.

Raising awareness of mental health issues is well known to be problematic and fraught with media hype. To bend the ear of politicians it seems it is necessary to swing between sensationalism or hard RCT-dominated scientific evidence. Therefore, mental health policy is derived from these two positions, both of which are extreme and of little application to the general population. To summarize then, the peer-review process, as determined by the publication process highlighted here, not only reports on research that has been funded but also impacts upon future research funding and indeed also influences what topics (and therein treatments) are hot and which are not.

Benchmarking practice: its place in the hierarchy of evidence

As systematic reviews and meta-analytic studies are held at being top of the hierarchy of evidence within the evidence-based practice paradigm, so benchmarking can be viewed as being an equivalently highly valued level of evidence within the practice-based paradigm. Therefore this second example of context will be given consideration in the remainder of this chapter. Benchmarking refers to the establishment of reference points that can be used to interpret data and in so doing to rate an organization in terms of quality indicators. Benchmarking is a highly complex practice. As observed in

Cahill et al. (2006), benchmarks are context dependent and need to be responsive to the research question, practitioners' needs, and constraints of service environment. In benchmarking practice there must be scrupulous attention to benchmark selection and appropriateness of use. Benchmarks derive from a context in which science in the form of measurement serves practice, meaning that there is significant potential for research to serve the needs of practice. However, it is important to keep certain caveats in mind. Firstly, developing benchmarks involves considerable data collection and a substantive infrastructure to achieve sizeable numbers of clients within a service and also a sizeable number of services. Secondly, although benchmarks initially appear to be precise, the large confidence intervals associated with the majority of benchmarks mean that the figures need to be interpreted with some caution (the confidence interval is the range within which the true treatment effect is likely to lie; Davies & Crombie, 2009). Finally, benchmarks are a more useful tool when considered over a period of time rather than as a one-off assessment meaning again that considerable infrastructure is needed which will necessarily incur considerable expense.

Many patients seek and access support for their mental health symptoms and concerns through primary health care, this is usually the first point of contact. Availability of therapeutic interventions varies across geographical regions, countries, and cultures. However, there has been an upsurge in the provision of short-term therapeutic interventions within general practice and primary care of late, namely, Cognitive-Behavioral Psychotherapy and short-term Psychodynamic Psychotherapy.

We cite three areas relating to research in such clinically representative settings that have been addressed by benchmarking and which we believe are significant determinants of practice:

(1) assessment outcomes
(2) equivalence of Psychodynamic Interpersonal Therapy (PIT) and Cognitive-Behavioral Therapy (CBT) within routine practice
(3) effectiveness of psychological therapies in routine settings as measured against efficacy benchmarks.

Assessment outcomes, defined by the Clinical Outcomes in Routine Evaluation Outcome Measure (CORE-OM) as the range of outcomes for the client following their assessment prior to therapy, are of significance to clinical practice in that they represent the client's experience of seeking therapy and mark the beginning of the therapeutic journey. The *equivalence of therapies*, likened to the dodo verdict in psychological literature (Everybody has won, and all must have prizes), has long been debated and vigorously contested in psychotherapy and counseling. Most recently, Stiles et al. (2008) provided support for the equivalence of treatments in routine settings—this publication attracted a great deal of controversy (e.g., Clark et al., 2008) indicating that the question of equivalence of outcomes in practice is strikingly pertinent and emotive to practitioners and educators alike. With regard to the *effectiveness of psychological therapies in routine settings*, benchmarking practice can be usefully employed to put clinically representative research on the map and to indicate differences and similarities within routine settings.

Interpreting the evidence

Assessment outcomes

In an analysis of 34 primary care services, it was found that a mean of 81% of clients were accepted into therapy, with significant variation among services ranging from 34% at the lower limit to 100% at the upper limit (Cahill et al., 2006). Such variation flags up ethical considerations in terms of a real possibility that large numbers of clients in some services have a negative experience of seeking therapy. However, we would emphasize that *assessment outcomes* derived from benchmarking exercises are context dependent and context bound. Particularly with *assessment outcomes*, there was a range of contextual factors influencing proportion of clients taken up for therapy such as availability of alternative services, waiting times, population demographics, commissioner expectations, and referrer pressures to take "hard to help" clients.

Equivalence of PIT and CBT in routine settings

Paley et al. (2008), in benchmarking against other studies conducted in routine settings, found that PIT was comparable with results of other therapies (including CBT) in routine settings. The authors concluded that this finding provides a degree of support for broad equivalence of outcomes in routine settings as observed by Stiles et al. (2008).

Effectiveness of therapies in routine settings benchmarked against therapies in efficacy studies

In benchmarking outcome data from a study examining the effectiveness of Cognitive Therapy (CT) in a clinically representative setting (Cahill et al., 2003) against data from *efficacy* research, support was provided for a trend consistent with clinical lore and evidence-based practice (EBP) wisdom: effects observed in efficacy trials tend to be attenuated when transferred to real world settings. Accordingly Cahill et al. (2003) observed that the pre–post effect sizes (ESs) for CT were lower than those observed in efficacy RCTs by about 0.7. This finding has been confirmed by other benchmarking studies. That is, Paley et al. (2008) found that the ESs from PIT as practiced in routine setting were less favorable than when used in efficacy trials. Moreover, Cahill et al. (2009) provided evidence of reduced effectiveness of therapy in routine settings in a systematic review of practice-based research on psychological therapies. When benchmarked against efficacy studies, practice-based studies yielded ESs that fell short of the selected benchmark. Finally, in an examination of sudden gains in therapy (Hardy et al., 2005), it was observed that the sudden gains (large reductions in symptom intensity between two sessions) observed in routine practice were more attenuated, more erratic, and less stable than those observed in efficacy trials.

Implications of benchmarking practice for mental health practice

The matter of context raises pressing methodological questions concerning how these benchmarks are produced and interpreted, and how such evidence, derived from benchmarking, contributes to the knowledge base of clinically representative research and influences clinical practice. Responsible reading of benchmarks, accompanied with a degree of reflection, has potential to lead to an approach that is responsive to context. For example, regarding the proportion of clients accepted into therapy, Cahill et al. (2006) note that a high level of clients accepted into therapy might indicate a high level of appropriate referral, or it could mean that the service is being uncritical in determining which clients are suitable for therapy. It is only knowledge of practitioner and service parameters that can result in appropriate measurement against benchmarks.

While these publications converge in demonstration of superior outcomes observed in *efficacy* research, they also raise questions pertinent to the establishment of clinically representative research as a unique paradigm and the politics of reading outcomes from clinical practice. So, while publications such as Cahill et al. (2003), Hardy et al. (2005), and Paley et al. (2008) provide evidence of therapies' reduced effectiveness in clinically representative settings, we would also, following Shadish et al. (2000), underline important differences between research agendas of *efficacy* research and clinically representative research and the implications this has for making sense of the outcomes. The practice of benchmarking clinically representative research against *efficacy* trials, while on one level appearing to confirm the hierarchy of evidence, also draws attention to the issue of responsiveness in the reading of the results. That is, to differences in design issues in clinical trials and natural settings such as inclusion and exclusion criteria, client heterogeneity, therapist differences: information that is essential for framing the reading of therapeutic outcomes and hence determining the effectiveness of practice.

Moving away from comparisons with *efficacy* research to comparisons *within* clinically representative research reveals other issues relevant to methodology and theories about therapy effectiveness. For example, Paley et al. (2008), in benchmarking against other clinically representative studies, found that PIT was comparable with results of other therapies (including CBT) in routine settings. We concluded that this finding provides a degree of support for broad equivalence of outcomes in routine settings as observed by Stiles et al. (2008). What does equivalence of outcomes indicate? One explanation could be the importance of common factors in routine settings. Put another way, do treatment-specific effects become more attenuated in routine settings? One argument could be that in routine settings where therapists do not practice under constraints observed in RCTs, equivalent outcomes indicate therapists' responsiveness to clients in the context of the unfolding therapeutic relationship rather than adherence to any specific model.

Similarly, the observation of Hardy et al. (2005) of sudden gains across a variety of treatment approaches in routine settings, albeit in less stable form, could also be indicative of trans-theoretical processes taking place in psychotherapy, such as therapist responsiveness to client interpersonal styles, client assimilation of problems over psychotherapy (see Stiles et al., 1990), and developments and ruptures in the therapeutic relationship. Hence, an interesting question for clinical practice is whether a decrease in design and methodology constraints in routine settings provides a context in which transtheoretical processes become more dominant.

Summary of how the different contexts of reviewing and benchmarking practices impact on mental health and practice environments

We have suggested previously that there is a symmetry between these two "contexts": while systematic reviews and meta-analytic studies are held at being top of the hierarchy of evidence within the evidence-based practice paradigm, so benchmarking can be viewed as being an equivalently highly valued level of evidence within the practice-based paradigm. So both "contexts" occupy a privileged and powerful position in the hierarchy of evidence and, as such, have potential to politicize knowledge production. In this sense they are an undeniably influential contextual factor for all practitioners appraising and implementing evidence in mental health care settings. What we hope we have highlighted is that, given these two "contexts" have privileged positions, there is also great scope for the same "contexts" to be employed with responsibility and integrity as methodological tools to ensure that research can best serve the needs of practice. So using our experience of conducting a review of peer-reviewed material from the JPMHN we have highlighted how findings, based on peer-reviewed material, have potential to favor some mental health treatments over others, and have implications for future research activity and subsequently treatments for further investment. And in terms of the effect on the practitioner and researcher, certain theoretical models will be supported with other more creative, contentious, or polemic models marginalized and isolated. So we hope we have cultivated an awareness of how evidence can be misconstrued if the practice of reviewing and peer reviewing is not undertaken responsibly, and the importance of ensuring that the practice of reviewing adheres to evidence-based models in being transparent and replicable. Similarly, benchmarking techniques are also open to misuse and we highlight the consideration that needs to be given to the clinical context in which the benchmarked outcomes are produced, namely knowledge of practitioner and service parameters that can result in appropriate measurement against benchmarks. So responsible reading of benchmarks and review practice, accompanied with a degree of reflection, has potential to lead to an approach that is responsive to context and beneficial to practice.

Concluding comments

Mental illness is not remarkable in the current global context; what is amazing is people's ability to maintain some sense of mental health. Furthermore, what is interesting is that it is not studied in any great depth. Everyday and ordinary practice is often taken for granted in this way, so making the ordinary extraordinary is a challenge to all practitioners. Can the sane be distinguished from the insane is a question that has faced researchers, judges, psychiatrists, the criminal justice system, and the like. Moreover such questions as: "Do the salient characteristics that lead to diagnoses (of mental illness) reside in the patients themselves or in the environment and contexts in which the observers find them?" raised by Rosenhan (2001, p. 70), continue to be debated.

"Symptoms" of mental illness can be reframed as offences against implicit understandings of particular cultures. Offences against norms carry conventional names; for example, an offence against property is called theft. There are however certain offences that belie conventional categorizations. Scheff (2001) gives the example of having a conversation with a colleague whilst scrutinizing their ear as opposed to looking at their face or into their eyes. He points out that these offences are placed into a residual catch-all category, for the convenience of society. He goes on to observe that "In earlier societies, the residual category was witchcraft, spirit possession or possession by the devil; today, it is mental illness. The symptoms of mental illness are, therefore, violations of residual rules" (2001, p. 65).

In a different context different rules apply, so take the same behavior and locate it within an institution known as the academy and the behavior is seen to be normal. The same could be said of research and evidence; any research that falls outside a traditional route has traditionally fallen into the residual category, although this is changing now. Which is of particular note for research and evidence in mental health as not only are the stereotypes of insanity continually reaffirmed, albeit inadvertently, in ordinary social interaction, but they are also perpetuated by research that does not take seriously the experience of the user. In the context of this book, that is you the reader. What we hope to have highlighted here are some of the ways in which the taken-for-granted assumptions around evidence can, and do, impact upon practice. We challenge practitioners, educators, and researchers alike to reflect on ways in which they can contribute to raising awareness of the importance of using and applying constructed wisdom both within and drawn from clinical practice.

References

Amin, M. & Mabe, M. (2000). Impact factors: Use and abuse. Retrieved October 29, 2009, from http://www.formatex.org/amvilas/impact.pdf.

Belenky, M., Clinchy, B., Goldbeger, N. & Tarule, J. (1986). Women's ways of knowing. New York: Basic Books.

Bishop, V. (2004). Knocking down the ivory towers: Publish and be damned. In: Freshwater, D. & Bishop, V. (eds) *Nursing Research in Context: Appreciation, Application and Professional Development.* Basingstoke: Palgrave, Chapter 10, pp. 168–187.

Cahill, J., Barkham, M., Hardy, G.E. et al. (2003). Outcomes of patients completing and not completing cognitive therapy for depression. *British Journal of Clinical Psychology,* 42(2), 133–143.

Cahill, J., Potter, S. & Mullin, T. (2006). First contact session outcomes in primary care psychological therapy and counselling services. *Counselling & Psychotherapy Research,* 6(1), 41–49.

Cahill, J., Barkham, M. & Stiles, W.B. (2009). Systematic review of practice-based research on psychological therapies in routine clinic settings. *British Journal of Clinical Psychology* [epub ahead of print].

Clark, D.M., Fairburn, C.G. & Wessely, S. (2008). Psychological treatment outcomes in routine NHS services: A commentary on Stiles et al. (2007). *Psychological Medicine* 38(5), 629–634.

Crosland, A. & Kai, J. (1998). "They think they can talk to nurses": practice nurses' views of their roles in caring for mental health problems. *British Journal of General Practice,* 48(432), 1383–1386.

Davies, H.T. & Crombie, I.K. (2009). What are confidence intervals and p-values? What is...? series. Available at http://www.medicine.ox.ac.uk/bandolier/painres/download/whatis/What_are_Conf_Inter.pdf (accessed November 8, 2009).

Davis, B.D. (1981). Trends in psychiatric nursing research. Occasional Paper, *Nursing Times,* 77, 73–76.

Freshwater, D. (2003). Pathology in a post modern society. *NTResearch* (now *Journal Research in Nursing*), 8(3), 161–172.

Freshwater, D. (ed.) (2005). Editorial: Re-viewing (A year in the life). *Journal of Psychiatric and Mental Health Nursing,* 12, 385–386.

Freshwater, D. (2007). Discourse, responsible research and positioning the subject. *Journal of Psychiatric and Mental Health Nursing,* 14(2), 111–112.

Freshwater, D. & Stickley, T. (2007). Emotional intelligence in mental health education. In: Stickley, T. & Basset, T. (eds) *Teaching Mental Health.* Chichester: Wiley, Chapter 13, pp. 161–170.

Hardy, G.E., Cahill, J., Stiles, W.B., Ispan, C., Macaskill, N. & Barkham, M. (2005). Sudden gains in cognitive therapy for depression: A replication and extension. *Journal of Consulting and Clinical Psychology,* 73(1), 59–67.

Jones, S.L. & Jones, P.K. (1987). Research in psychiatric and mental health nursing: The emergence of scientific rigor. *Archives of Psychiatric Nursing*, 1(3), 155–162.

Merwin, E. & Mauck, A. (1995). Psychiatric nursing outcome research: The state of the science. *Archives of Psychiatric Nursing*, 9, 311–331.

O'Toole, A.W. (1981). When the theoretical becomes practical. *Journal of Psychosocial Nursing and Mental Health Services*, 19, 11–19.

Paley, G., Cahill, J., Barkham, M. et al. (2008). The effectiveness of psychodynamic–interpersonal psychotherapy in routine clinical practice: A benchmarking comparison. *Psychology and Psychotherapy: Theory, Research and Practice*, 81(2), 157–175.

Parry, G. (1996). Using research to change practice. In: Heller, T., Reynolds, J., Gomm, J., Muston, R. & Pattison, S. (eds) *Mental Health Matters: A Reader*. Basingstoke: Palgrave, Chapter 34.

Rosenhan, D.L. (2001). On being sane in insane places. In: Heller, T., Reynolds, J., Gomm, J., Muston, R. & Pattison, S. (eds) *Mental Health Matters: A Reader*. Basingstoke: Palgrave, Chapter 9.

Shadish, W.R., Navarro, A.M., Matt, G.E. & Phillips, G. (2000). The effects of psychological therapies under clinically representative conditions: A meta-analysis. *Psychological Bulletin*, 126, 512–529.

Scheff, T.J. (2001). Labelling mental illness. In: Heller, T., Reynolds, J., Gomm, J., Muston, R. & Pattison, S. (eds) *Mental Health Matters: A Reader*. Basingstoke: Palgrave, Chapter 8.

Stiles, W.B., Elliot, R., Llewelyn, S.P. et al. (1990). Assimilation of problematic experiences by clients in psychotherapy. *Psychotherapy*, 27, 411–420.

Stiles, W.B., Barkham, M., Mellor-Clark, J. & Connell, J. (2008). Effectiveness of cognitive-behavioural, person-centred, and psychodynamic therapies in UK primary-care routine practice: Replication in a larger sample. *Psychological Medicine*, 38, 677–688.

Ward, A. (2008). Psychological therapies provision: Views from primary care. *Psychiatric Bulletin*, 32, 369–374.

Yonge, O., Austin, W., Zhou Qiuping, P., Wacko, M., Wilson, S. & Zaleski, J. (1997). A systematic review of the psychiatric/mental health nursing research literature 1982–1992. *Journal of Psychiatric and Mental Health Nursing*, 4, 171–177.

Chapter 9

Making context work in aged care

Nadine Janes

Introduction

It is timely to examine how to provide the best in healthcare for older persons. People are living longer and healthier lives around the world. It has been projected that 20% of the world's population will be aged 60 years or older by the year 2050 (WHO, 2003). As much as one third of the population in some countries including Greece, Italy, Japan, Korea, and Spain will be aged 65 and over by the same year (OECD, 2007). In keeping with the current mandate for evidence-based practice, strategies are needed to ensure that the healthcare provided to the growing number of older persons is grounded in the best available knowledge. Unfortunately, a lack of empirical attention specific to evidence-based practices within the context of aged care settings has left us poorly informed about what those strategies might be.

This chapter explores evidence-based practice within the discrete context of institutional aged care. Long-term care (LTC) homes as a primary aged care setting will be highlighted as unique from other healthcare institutions in relation to the staff mix and educational preparation, the clinical needs of residents, and the overall focus of care. Key findings from an evolving program of research will shed light on what might influence the evidence-based nature of the care provided in LTC homes given these contextual variables. The findings are based on the integrated perspectives of unregulated care providers who work in LTC homes and of facilitators of evidence-based practice within these settings. What will be revealed is the significant influence of the leadership, as well as the overall relational dynamics within LTC homes. Furthermore, the personal traits of formal care providers on an emotional as well as intellectual level warrant particular attention if goals to promote better institutional aged care are to be fully realized.

Aged care settings and providers

Healthcare for older persons is provided across a range of settings. Hospitals provide temporary, episodic services for older persons when they are acutely ill. The focus of such services is on curing illness in the shortest period of time in keeping with an established trend across the globe to decrease acute care stays and provide the majority of healthcare in the community. When an older person is recovering from an acute illness or is chronically ill, there is generally a continuum of care services and settings available in the community to provide healthcare with a focus on minimizing, rehabilitating, or compensating for losses of independent physical and/or mental functioning. The extent of this service provision may vary from country to country.

The continuum of community-based options begins with home, which is widely considered the best place to provide care. A range of services exist in varying degrees in many countries to help sustain and/or supplement the informal care contributions provided by family members and to enable older persons to live in their homes for as long as possible. In Ontario, Canada, these services include assistance with homemaking, security checks/telephone assurance programs, home maintenance and repair, delivery of meals, foot care, friendly visiting, transportation to essential appointments, and personal care assistance (e.g., bathing, dressing) (Ontario Seniors' Secretariat, 2007). Family members might also elect to access respite care to support their caregiving efforts, a particular community-based service aimed at providing informal care providers with "time off" from their caregiving. It may be provided within the home by a formal care provider, through an adult day program in a community or healthcare center, or in a residential healthcare institution through short-stay programs. Older persons admitted into short-stay respite beds within institutions are expected to return to their home in the community within a specified period of time.

Changes to family as an institution are leading to a reduced ability of families to care for aging members with chronic conditions in the home regardless of what community services are available for supplemental support (OECD, 2005). These changes include declining birthrates as well as the migration of young people from rural to urban areas, and from poorer to richer countries. Furthermore, women, the traditional caregivers in society, are increasingly less available for the role as they are pulled to external employment by economic necessity or personal desire (WHO, 2003). The capabilities of families to meet the healthcare needs of their older relatives are particularly challenged when the individual is suffering from a chronic dementing disorder such as Alzheimer's disease or a related dementia (ADRD). With the growing global population of older persons comes an increase in diseases associated with aging such as ADRD, which afflicts 11% of those aged 75–84 and as many as 35% of persons 85 and older (Alzheimer's Disease International, 2009). While community-based services may initially be sufficient to support families in meeting the care needs of older persons with ADRD, by the later phases of the illness they are often insufficient for meeting the afflicted person's inevitable need for continuous care. Admission of older persons to a residential setting for accommodation and care eventually becomes a reality for many families. Retirement homes (i.e., rest homes) provide minimal to moderate support with daily living activities, while LTC homes (i.e., nursing homes, residential care homes, skilled nursing facilities) provide 24-h nursing and personal care. A WHO study estimated that, in many developing countries, the need for care in LTC homes in particular will increase by as much as 400% in the coming decades (WHO, 2003).

LTC homes provide for an older person's socialization as well as healthcare needs on a continuous basis. Countries differ widely in the privacy and amenities available to residents in these settings (OECD, 2005). The nursing and personal care offered are supplemented by varying levels of recreational activities, therapy services, counseling, and spiritual care. In contrast to the medical model underpinning acute care in hospitals, the focus of activities in LTC homes is to promote quality of life and optimize residents' independent functioning, despite the presence of disability, for as long as possible. LTC homes are also distinct from acute care settings in relation to the skill mix of nursing staff and the clinical nature of the resident population.

Beyond acute care institutions, unregulated care providers (UCPs, e.g., certified nursing assistants, home health aides, home care workers, healthcare aides, and personal support workers) represent the primary providers of formal aged care. They provide the majority of low intensity personal care as well as have the most direct continuing contact with older persons, and are therefore essential to helping older persons with care needs maintain quality in their later life. In LTC homes, UCPs are the primary providers of direct hands-on care including assistance with bathing, dressing, toileting, and meals. In Ontario, they provide 75% of such care, while Registered Nurses (RNs) within LTC homes focus more on decision making, analysis, critical thinking, and leadership among other care providers (OANHSS, 1998). In the absence of the medical resources and technical support available within acute care settings, the RN in LTC is needed to coordinate and direct care for residents who experience complex and unpredictable conditions. The RN role also includes providing hands-on guidance and supervision of UCP practice, as well as troubleshooting for service provision issues in the residential care area. When Registered Practical Nurses (i.e., RPNs, Licensed Practical Nurses in some jurisdictions, Enrolled Nurses in the UK, Australia, and New Zealand) are part of the skill mix, they support the work of the RN by contributing to the assessment of residents, the guidance and support of UCPs, and the administration of medications and treatments.

The formal training of UCPs is minimal, currently standardized at only 500 h in the province of Ontario—225 h theory (classroom), 10 h evaluation, and 265 h practicum (work placement) (OCS Association, 1997—reissued 2009). This standard is beyond the quantity of learning provided in other countries and jurisdictions. The fit of UCPs' level of education with the care needs of residents in today's LTC homes is questionable and has been cited as a primary concern of long-term care policy makers across a number of countries (OECD, 2005). Residents in LTC homes are increasingly more frail and complex, due to the shorter lengths of stay in acute care settings and the transfer of much healthcare to community settings described earlier. Furthermore, their care needs are complex by virtue of the fact that many are living with ADRD, also referred to earlier. Older persons with ADRD account for the majority of residents in LTC homes rising to as high as 90% of the resident population in several countries, suggesting that such facilities have become "insidiously specialized in AD disease" (Moise et al., 2004, p. 82).

People with ADRD suffer progressive cognitive and functional losses that ultimately render them incapable of independently meeting even their most basic of activities of daily living. Additionally, many will display distressing symptoms at various phases of their illness including verbal and/or physical aggression, socially inappropriate behavior, wandering, or resistance to care. Some countries including Great Britain, Germany, Sweden, the USA, and Canada single out persons with ADRD for care on specialized units within LTC homes (Moise et al., 2004). These special care units (SCUs) provide for the needs of the most complex and challenging of residents with ADRD while remaining units provide for the needs of persons with ADRD who are manageable within an integrated care setting where persons without cognitive impairment also reside. When a facility does not have a SCU, all persons with ADRD, regardless of their care or behavioral profiles, live alongside residents without dementia.

Providing care to older persons with ADRD is physically and emotionally exhausting. Although in theory the registered nursing staff (i.e., RNs and RPNs) within LTC homes are meant to aid UCPs in managing their care responsibilities, their workloads prohibit them from providing a prompt response to every resident care situation and from providing continuous consultation and support to UCPs who are also burdened by low staff:resident ratios. A case in point is the expectation placed on RNs in some Ontario LTC homes to be responsible for the care of 200 or more residents (ONA, 2007). Concerns over the workload of registered nursing staff in LTC homes have been cited elsewhere (Karlsson et al., 2008). UCPs are consequently left to function with minimal instruction at a relatively independent level and to apply their knowledge and problem solve as needed during caregiving despite the practice complexities and challenges they face.

Best practice in aged care

Indeed LTC homes are unique in relation to the composite of nursing staff and the clinical needs of residents, the majority of whom live with a chronic dementia. The overall focus of care is also distinct in its divergence from the curative medical model so pervasive in prominent healthcare settings such as acute care. These contextual elements of LTC contribute to a final unique aspect of aged care in these settings and that is the nature of the knowledge that is required by formal care providers such as UCPs to meet their caregiving responsibilities. Promoting evidence-based practice in LTC does not require the dissemination and facilitated uptake and use of highly technical instrumental knowledge. Rather, the "evidence" that is needed to promote better care is predominantly conceptual in nature. Key to best care practices in LTC is the UCPs' use of knowledge about ways of relating with older persons, such that they feel secure, able, and valued as unique human beings. These interpersonal patterns represent a shift from traditional routinized and custodial approaches to the care of older persons. While not highly technical and instrumental in nature, these patterns are nonetheless challenging to accomplish given the declining cognitive and functional capacities of LTC residents.

Person-centered care (McCormack, 2004; Tellis-Nayak, 2007), individualized care (Chappell et al., 2006; Cohen-Mansfield, 2000), and relationship-based care (McGilton, 2002) are frameworks that have been used to organize conceptual knowledge about best aged care approaches in general, and about dementia care specifically. Rather than providing a standard, concrete protocol to guide one's practice, such knowledge suggests how one should think about older persons as well as the care provider role. Cohen-Mansfield and Purpura-Gill (2008, p. 378) characterized quality practice styles in LTC homes as those that demonstrate "respect for the resident as a person, compassion for the resident's position, promotion of self-determination whenever possible, individualization of care to match a resident's characteristics, and maximization of comfort and contentment." These relational styles reflect a welcome alternative to the dehumanization so often associated with experiences as patients in today's high-tech, fast-paced healthcare system. However, expressed concern in the literature about deficiencies in the quality of aged care within LTC homes indicates that such practices have yet to be universally realized (Caspar & O'Rourke, 2008; Cohen-Mansfield & Purpura-Gill, 2008; Owen, 2008; Teeri et al., 2008).

A program of research on evidence-based aged care

The quality of care of institutionalized older persons in LTC homes is largely dependent on the ability of UCPs, as the primary care providers, to utilize best practice knowledge in the context of their day-to-day practice responsibilities. What UCPs do and how they do it have the potential to mitigate residents' suffering associated with the progressive loss of their functional and/or cognitive capacities as a result of chronic conditions such as ADRD. Literature related to evidence-based healthcare practice to-date is of limited use in promoting best aged care because of its predominant focus on the practice of professional care providers (e.g., RNs) and on instrumental knowledge use in acute care settings.

We do not, as yet, know how the context of LTC homes, as described above, relates to the presence or absence of evidence-based practice within these facilities. A program of research was initiated to help fill this knowledge gap and build foundational understanding about evidence-based practice in a priority aged care context. The initial study involved grounded theory method to build a middle range theory of the process by which UCPs utilize knowledge about person-centered care in dementia care settings. Data were collected through face-to-face interviews with 20 UCPs working in SCUs across 8 urban LTC homes in Toronto, Canada. Residents of these 32-bed SCUs had a diagnosis of ADRD, were at risk of eloping from the facility, and/or displayed disruptive and complex behaviors.

The theory was refined and validated through a second investigation involving focus group methodology. Twenty UCPs working in a 500-bed rural LTC home outside of Toronto, Canada, participated in serial focus groups during which time they were presented with the original theory of knowledge utilization and asked to clarify, elaborate, and validate the theory's underlying concepts. The UCPs in this second study worked either on the facility's SCU or on a regular unit so as to broaden the applicability of the theory to the practice of UCPs caring for older persons with ADRD across all units within a LTC home. The demographics of participants for the initial two studies are described in Table 9.1.

A third study was conducted to elicit the perspective of facilitators of knowledge utilization in LTC homes about the factors that influence their work. Descriptions of critical incidents from the day-to-day practice of 34 professionals responsible for encouraging nursing staffs' utilization of best practice knowledge in LTC homes within the province of Ontario were collected through face-to-face interviews, telephone interviews, and a written questionnaire on a secured web site. A total of 123 critical incidents about facilitators' frustrations and satisfactions were analyzed to reveal a list of factors that impact on their success in enhancing the evidence-based nature of nursing practice, including that of UCPs, within LTC homes.

Table 9.1 Unregulated care provider participant demographics

Demographic	Grounded theory study (N = 20)	Focus group study (N = 20) (SCU = 5; LTC unit = 15)
Gender	Male = 3; Female = 17	Male = 1; Female = 19
Age (years)	<31 = 0; 31–50 = 9; >50 = 11	<31 = 2; 31–50 = 12; >50 = 6
Employment status	FT = 12; PT = 8	FT = 7; PT = 13
Shift	D = 7; E = 6; D/E = 7	D = 10; E = 0; D/E = 10
Work experience—current (years)	<5 = 6; 5–10 = 1; 11–16 = 7; >17 = 6	<5 = 6; 5–10 = 4; 11–16 = 3; >17 = 3; no response = 4
Healthcare education*	None = 1; UCP = 19; Other = 8	None = 0; UCP = 20; Other = 1
Country of origin	Canada = 1; Other = 19	Canada = 10; Other = 10

SCU, special care unit; LTC, long-term care; FT, full time; PT, part-time; D, day shift; E, evening shift; D/E, day and evening shifts.
*UCP—formal training as an unregulated care provider.

Table 9.2 Facilitator participant demographics

Demographic	N
Age	Range = 28–62 years; Median = 49 years
Gender	Male = 2; Female = 32
Ethnicity*	Caucasian = 29; Other = 2
Highest education*	C = 5; UU = 15; GU = 11
Years worked present facilitator role	Range = 0–7 years; Median = 4.25 years
Years worked prior facilitator role(s)	Range = 0–16 years; Median = 3 years
Employment status*	FT = 30; PT = 3
Scope of practice*,†	Range = 1–79; Median = 11 homes
Percentage facilitator role*,‡	Range = 10–85; Median = 50

C, college; UU, undergraduate university degree; GU, graduate university degree; FT, full time; PT, part-time.
*Some data are missing for this demographic.
†Number of LTC homes within responsibilities.
‡Percentage of work time spent in facilitator activities.

While facilitators were not asked to focus specifically on their efforts to enhance the utilization of person-centered care in the context of dementia care, 79 (64%) incidents were thus focused. The demographics of the participants for this study are described in Table 9.2.

It is beyond the scope of this chapter to detail all findings from the three studies which have in part been reported elsewhere (Janes et al., 2008, 2009). Rather, a narrative summary of select themes that reflect the most common threads across the data is presented. Provided is a précis of what influences the evidence-based nature of aged care within the practice context of LTC homes—a setting where UCPs assume primary responsibility for the hands-on care of complex and frail older people, most of whom have ADRD, without having benefited from extensive educational preparation or without having timely and consistent guidance from registered nursing staff. Direct quotes from the first two studies will have a superscript "UCP" to identify the source of the data (i.e., unregulated care providers). The superscript "F" will be used to make clear which data resulted from the critical incident study involving the perspective of facilitators of best aged care practice. Findings from the literature are embedded throughout the narrative to illustrate parallels between the data from the studies reported here and evolving understandings of UCP practice in LTC.

Influences on evidence-based aged care

It would be reasonable to assume that a common complaint of UCPs and facilitators of evidence-based practice alike in LTC homes would be that insufficient staff, unrealistic workloads, and a lack of time are primarily responsible for a lack of best practice in caregiving. These organizational concerns in relation to LTC homes have been well documented (Fläckman et al., 2008). However, while cited by a number of UCP and facilitator participants across the studies reported here, these factors did not surface as the most influential in the particular context of evidence-based practice. As one participant explained, *I think we don't complain a lot about the time because we know there's nothing we can do about that and so we tend to focus on the things we can do something about*[UCP]. The absence of workload factors in the following descriptions should not undermine the very real challenges associated with minimal staffing patterns in relation to quality in healthcare. Rather, the descriptions perhaps should be interpreted as a reflection of what the chosen categories of participants (i.e., UCPs and facilitators) perceived as more amenable to improvement and, therefore, important for others to hear in the interest of enhancing the evidence-based nature of aged care in LTC homes.

Being a formal caregiver in LTC homes is not without its difficulties: *I think it can go from one end of the spectrum to the other. It's frustrating some days and it's a lot of fun other days*[UCP]. UCPs identified clinical factors related to dementia care as particularly challenging, namely, the unpredictable, variable, and aggressive behaviors of older persons with ADRD labeled as *the game of chance*[UCP] and *the fighting spirit*[UCP], respectively. In terms of the former, UCP participants were aware of the uniqueness of residents and struggled at times with the variable and changeable ways that they respond to caregiving.

Studies have indicated that aggressive resident behaviors are prevalent and stressful for nursing caregivers in dementia care practice in LTC settings (McPhaul & Lipscomb, 2004; Skovdahl et al., 2003). Parallel findings echoed in the data from all UCP participants as they recounted numerous situations of actual or anticipated aggressive resident behaviors:

> I remember being grabbed one night . . . and I could swear I could hear the bones in my wrist crunching. This guy had me . . . by both wrists and he's got me like this and he wasn't pushing or anything, he was just squeezing and this man had the biggest hands and I swear I could hear the bones crunching and I was just like, and I was trying to talk to him very calmly. Inside I was terrified[UCP].

The extent to which UCPs are able to use conceptual knowledge about best aged care practices, given the *game of chance* and the *fighting spirit* that typify the clinical context of LTC, is influenced largely by the relational tone of a facility and by a UCP's personal capacities on both emotional and intellectual levels. In regard to the relational tone, the nature of interpersonal patterns between UCPs and administrative leaders as well as registered nursing staff and residents' families were held largely responsible by study participants for how supportive or obstructive the tone was to best practice patterns.

Leadership: epicenter of change or root of resistance

Both UCP and facilitator participants alike across the three studies notably made an effort to reflect fairly on the complexities involved in promoting evidence-based aged care and the consequent err of pointing to any one person, process, or attribute of LTC settings as solely responsible for deficiencies in practice patterns. However, most suggested that one could not deny the pivotal role that administrative leaders (e.g., Director of Care, Managers) in LTC play in setting the conditions necessary for direct care providers to reach their potential for practice excellence. Conversely, it was suggested that they are equally capable of setting up blocks to knowledge transfer initiatives and perpetuating outdated and ineffective care practices. Olson and Zwygart-Stauffacher (2008) similarly suggested that Directors of Nursing, key administrative leaders within LTC, have the potential to greatly influence organizational performance in these settings. As one facilitator insisted,

> . . . we can train the front-line staff until the cows come home, but we will never see true paradigm shifts in long-term care until we work to support the leaders and managers of the home to transform the home itself. [best practice] comes from the top down, as well as from the bottom up[F].

Facilitators believed strongly that without overt managerial *support*[F], a practice enhancement initiative would fail. Management personnel were identified as having *the final say*[F] in regard to all evidence-based practice initiatives.

The nature of the relationship between administrative leaders and UCPs can influence the ultimate success of facilitators' efforts to promote evidence-based practice: . . . *if there are under currents of staff-management tensions, unrest, union problems, those sort of things, they can certainly interfere with creating a good culture of learning*[F]. Without exception facilitators highlighted the importance of helping manage relationships between management and staff to build their individual successes. Disheartening to many was their experience that, characteristically, negative relationships seemed deeply embedded in the culture of LTC homes and endemic across the sector:

> There is not enough understandable incentive . . . in fact there is disincentive . . . for the people who are paid so poorly and expected . . . and so much is expected of them. And so little given back to them. And I don't mean that as a blame to particular managers or anything. I think it's just an institutionalized set of relationships and behaviours[F].

Descriptions of disempowering leadership styles, where there is *great emphasis on control*[F], were detailed by UCPs and facilitators as the most contrary to the conditions needed for successful knowledge transfer at the point-of-care. These sentiments echo the links others have made between UCP empowerment and the nature of the care they provide to older persons in LTC (Bowers et al., 2003; Caspar & O'Rourke, 2008; Cready et al., 2008). A relational element lacking in disempowering leadership styles is recognition or reward for a job well done, which was identified by all UCP participants and explicitly linked to their motivation to strive toward practice excellence:

> In this line of work historically I have never had not even a manager or anyone say to me, what do you think? . . . and when these things happen, it gives you the courage you need and the people want to do more and more . . . those are the things that keep you going because somebody tells you thank you . . . respect from other people makes you apply yourself professionally[UCP].

Sustaining the ability to provide best aged care, given the unpredictable, variable, and threatening clinical nature of LTC homes where the majority of residents have ADRD, is difficult. It requires that a care provider reach out to a resident, relate with warmth and patience, and ensure that the resident is made to feel safe and cared for. These expectations exist despite the fact that residents may counter such efforts with resistance and aggressive behavior (i.e., *fighting spirit*). Such tensions are unique to the LTC practice context and may provide some explanation why UCPs are so in need of recognition for their caregiving efforts. Facilitator participants were particularly attuned to the link between appreciation and a UCP's ultimate readiness to learn and use best practice knowledge:

> My emotional outlook toward the staff is very important. When I am talking to them, I consciously try to feel emotionally supportive and caring about them . . . I believe that if we want staff to care about the residents, then we have to care about the staff. I believe that when a person feels cared about, it gives them the strength to apply this caring approach on to others that they care for...[F]

Facilitators worked to motivate nursing staff in general toward evidence-based practice by offering them *praise*[F] and acknowledging their *strengths*[F], *accomplishments*[F], and *efforts*[F] in regard to providing best care for their residents.

Social relations: harmony or autocracy

UCP participants suggested that regardless of what they thought would be "best" in a moment of practice, at times their decision making was subjugated to the wishes of others. Any suggestion that UCPs are always free to use best practice knowledge may reflect what has been referred to as the "autonomy bias" inherent in much of the evidence-based practice literature. Beyond the relationship between administrative leaders and UCPs already described, those amongst levels of nursing staff and with residents' families were high-lighted as particularly influential in regard to UCPs' use or nonuse of best practice knowledge.

Not unlike other healthcare settings LTC homes are inherently hierarchical. What is unique about the LTC context however, is the addition of UCPs to the hierarchy and in particular, their position-ing at the bottom: *Well a lot of them [registered staff] treat us like we're beneath them. And I'm sorry to say but it's the truth . . . We're on the bottom of the totem pole*[UCP]. According to UCPs, autocracy amongst the levels of nursing staff influences the evidence-based nature of practice through its impact on UCPs' ability to act on their knowledge of what might be best for residents:

> It's difficult as a [UCP] . . . we're not registered staff . . . So some-times we know what might help but what we say . . . Does not make a difference to the registered staff . . . because we are [UCPs] . . . They think we are lower than them . . . Any RN, RPN, we're the lower of the totem pole . . . We're actually the ones that do the care. You sit there and write it on paper . . . And no matter what theory we give them, they go with their own. Ours is not good enough for them . . . But we know because we do it and we do it every day[UCP].

Many facilitator participants affirmed these relational patterns labeled by one participant as UCPs being *put into a situation that they're between a rock and a hard place*[F] and having to go *against their better judgment*[F].

Just as UCP participants linked evidence-based practice to their relationships with RNs and RPNs, quality care for older people has been linked by others to the interrelationships between registered nursing staff and UCPs in LTC homes (Karlsson et al., 2008). In Karlsson and colleague's study, collaborative relationships, where

UCPs are respected for the knowledge they bring to resident care decision making, are more likely to lead to quality care practices. Facilitator participants highlighted the positive influence of registered staff relational styles that were *encouraging*[F], *enabling*[F], and *positive*[F]. Furthermore, facilitators themselves worked to provide opportunities for UCPs to exchange knowledge with other members of the healthcare team and to be valued by all for their contributions to resident care planning: *It's important that they have a voice because I find the frontline staff are the ones with the least voice and yet they are the ones that are providing that direct contact, so they like to share their ideas*[F].

Aside from interprofessional relations, discord between families of residents and nursing care providers in LTC homes has been cited (Lau et al., 2008). While UCP participants did describe some families in a positive light, many did speak about disharmony with families that may undermine a UCP's ability to make autonomous decisions about the use of best practice knowledge.

Older persons in LTC homes are admitted for the long term. This means that any involved family members they have become part of the relational fabric of the facility over time. Indeed UCP participants broadened the composite of the hierarchical structure within their workplace beyond the interrelationships amongst levels of nursing staff and administrators to include the positioning of residents' families. Universally they were represented by participants as another group above the UCP on the proverbial totem pole:

> . . . family somehow they don't see us as professional caregivers because they, I don't know the information that we are here like . . . We're servants in a hotel . . . do what we're told, ya, so we don't understand and we don't know better. And they treat us like, you know, not independent like basically people with[out] any knowledge really . . .[UCP]

As is the case with interprofessional relations, the positioning of families above UCPs influences evidence-based practice through its impact on a UCP's ability to do what they "know" is best for residents: *family has the final say*[UCP].

UCP participants viewed many families as being in *denial*[UCP] about their older relative's health condition or that they *need more education*[UCP] to better understand what the individual's care needs really are. Consequently, families at times place expectations on UCPs to provide care in ways that are not always consistent with best practice as understood by the UCPs. Most often, this was exemplified by UCPs feeling that they had to *force*^{UCP} personal care on their residents regardless of the means when combating the *fighting spirit*:

> They don't understand . . . A lot of them don't. I don't think they really understand the disease. They don't understand why that person, oh well "they were never like that" . . . It's acceptance. They don't want to accept . . . And you know when they're walking in the door it's stressful because they demand a lot . . . And you know "why is my mother's hair not combed?". And you know "I'm sorry but she runs her fingers through it a hundred times" . . . And you know "why is my mother's teeth dirty?" or "not in?". Well "she tried to bite me when I put them in" you know . . . ^{UCP}

The consequences of not using any means, best practice or not, to meet family expectations were clear to UCP participants and again related to the hierarchy within LTC—management becomes involved and workers get *dragged up on the carpet*^{UCP}.

UCP participants clearly linked hierarchical and dismissive relations within LTC to a lack of evidence-based practice. Conversely, harmonious and inclusive relations were explicitly tied to their ability to influence care provision in a positive way and to their motivation toward practice excellence. Characteristic of key strategies used by facilitators of better aged care practice is the explicit focus on flattening hierarchical relational patterns as well as promoting a greater sense of *camaraderie*^{F}, *teamwork*^{F}, *respect*^{F}, and *trust*^{F} within the LTC setting:

> Although I was facilitating these decisions and lending them my knowledge background they were part of the decision making process. I felt there was a sense of empowerment that they had made the decision versus being told what to do . . . the relationship developed is that they feel free to ask for advice and information without being judged on their knowledge level^F.

Caregiver quality: altruism or nihilism

Findings from all three studies suggest that evidence-based practice cannot be understood and promoted without considering the traits of the formal care providers who are being encouraged to transform their practice into better ways of relating to their residents. As repeatedly highlighted, LTC homes are unique in their staff complement in that UCPs represent the primary care providers. UCPs themselves and facilitator participants suggested that this category of worker poses particular challenges to facilitating better aged care by virtue of their emotional and intellectual traits, the former receiving the most emphasis across participant data and therefore comprising the majority of this discussion.

A number of UCP participants described some of their peers as having an unselfish regard for or devotion to the well being of residents, labeled by one UCP participant as *heart and soul*[UCP]. Facilitator participants affirmed the altruism of many UCPs, which ultimately contributed to successful knowledge transfer initiatives:

> Most staff I have worked with have a genuine care for their patients . . . we have great staff in the system! 99% are passionate, intelligent people who are in long-term care for all the right reasons. They believe in person-centred care and work to achieve it[F].

However, a number of participants across both categories expressed concern with staff who lack the *compassion*[UCP] and *openness to change*[F] deemed essential to sustaining efforts to provide best aged care to spite the stressors associated with LTC practice. Facilitator participants, in particular, described a *pervasive negativity*[F] and *therapeutic nihilism*[F] within some LTC homes and the inability of many staff to entertain the potential for better practice options:

> There seems to be a genuine unwillingness to change or even entertain the thought of change but place their efforts into complaining that nothing works, we've tried that, it didn't work[F].

Lipe and Beasley (2004) suggested that it is very difficult to make sound clinical decisions while experiencing extreme emotions. One can therefore understand the negative influence of UCP emotions such as *hostility*[F], *irritability*[F], *resentment*[F], and *hopelessness*[F], all witnessed by facilitator participants, on a UCP's ability to engage in the process of taking up and ultimately using best practice knowledge. Indeed one facilitator participant highlighted how *keeping emotions [of UCPs] manageable is needed before they are ready for learning*[F]. This was largely accomplished by facilitator efforts to provide opportunities for staff to express their feelings during informal practice discussions. They also personally endeavored to counter staff stress and negativity and to contribute to a positive emotional climate that fostered learning and professional growth. They purposefully displayed *enthusiasm*[F] and described their concerted efforts to stay *positive*[F] and *upbeat*[F] toward staff.

Many UCP participants demonstrated an awareness of the link between their emotions and their ability to engage in evidence-based practice. They identified the importance of maintaining their composure when the *game of chance* and the *fighting spirit* led to frustration and upset so as not to thwart their ability to think through what would be best to do in a moment of practice. Furthermore, they recognized how their emotional responses to caregiving challenges, when received by residents, have the potential to escalate already difficult situations and further complicate their ability to provide the best in care:

> You have to keep a level head . . . just the way it is . . . especially the special care . . . Well the residents pick up on stuff like that when you're stressed . . . They're very sensitive . . . because it may come across in your voice but you just may not notice it coming out . . . your tone of your voice . . . they pick up on stuff like that and it caused them to get more aggressive[UCP].

Unique to the LTC practice context is the residential status of older persons being cared for by UCPs. As a result superficiality in the care provider—care recipient relationship has the potential to give way to a deeper connection over time. This connection might inadvertently contribute to a UCP's negative emotionality. That is, a number of UCPs expressed heightened frustration or upset when recounting practice situations that involved residents for whom they cared deeply and which resulted in negative care outcomes:

> . . . we had a lady passed away now but she fought to the bitter end. I came out of that room crying so many times. Not because she kicked me or punched me or anything like that. It's because you're so frustrated . . . because you want to help this woman and you know she's demented. She had a lot of evil spirits in there, I'm telling you, and it just made you cry[UCP].

Emotions aside, evidence-based practice is dependent on a care provider's intellectual capacity for clinical decision making. A complete account of how UCPs in the first study described their decision-making process has been reported elsewhere (Janes et al., 2008). For purposes of this chapter, it is important to highlight that UCPs' minimal formal training leaves them lacking in both the depth of knowledge necessary for best aged care practices as well as the analytical thinking skills to contextualize best practice knowledge for specific caregiving moments and to transfer the knowledge across different clinical situations. A number of UCP participants revealed their struggles associated with their clinical decision making:

> And then whatever you learn at school, like it's like somewhere else ... you thinking, oh my gosh, what to do? What can I do? What's going to work right now? Should I give him a choice? Should I just go and bath? Or try and get him, you know? I have to get the job done or else management or whatever like they're going to come around ... That's right ... and it's all your fault. So, and one minute you are facing one thousand choices in your mind ...[UCP]

All UCPs may not readily embrace theoretical and empirical sources of knowledge: *most of it is, well scientific stuff and you can take that with a grain of salt[UCP]*. Facilitator participants indeed described their efforts to accommodate UCPs' preferred learning through experience and human sources of knowledge. They disseminated best practice knowledge to UCPs indirectly through bedside *discussions[F]* and *case-based learning[F]* strategies. They framed these discussions in ways that the knowledge would be more likely viewed by UCPs as *feasible[F]*, *relevant[F]*, and *meaningful[F]* to the *real world[F]* clinical challenges they face. Knowledge was furthermore translated by facilitators and presented in *concrete[F]* and ready-to-use formats for UCPs. These compensatory strategies were designed in specific consideration of the disconnect between UCPs' intellectual capacities and the complex care needs of their residents.

Summary: maximize relationships, minimize stress

The uniqueness of LTC homes as a healthcare setting is reflected in the use of UCPs as primary care providers, the prevalence of ADRD amongst residents, and the focus of services on maximizing residents' functioning and promoting quality of living in a residential context. Promoting evidence-based aged care, given these contextual factors, might best be accomplished through a focus on maximizing relationships and minimizing stressors. These efforts represent a divergence from traditional educational strategies that have widely been used alone to better the quality of care in LTC homes. They move beyond the notion that filling the heads of UCPs with knowledge will automatically translate into better action at the point-of-care. The connection between knowledge and action is much more complex, as revealed in the perspectives of UCPs and facilitators that have been described in this chapter; a complexity that is in part embedded in the relational and emotional undertones of a LTC home.

The process by which UCPs use best practice knowledge is largely social in nature. That is, UCPs draw on human sources of best practice knowledge; rely on positive social relations to motivate and emotionally equip them for using the knowledge; and face power differentials involving relations with management, registered nursing staff, and resident families that impact on their autonomous decision making about the knowledge. Relational factors have not received much-focused attention in the nursing literature related to evidence-based practice nor have they been subjected to systematic investigation. In contrast, UCP and facilitator participants, from my research, identified relational factors as remarkably influential in the process by which best practice knowledge gets utilized in LTC homes. Current international literature related to care practices in LTC homes has highlighted the impact of social and political relations on the quality of UCPs' work experiences (Bowers et al., 2003; Cready et al., 2008; Fläckman et al., 2008; Robinson & Tappen, 2008). The practices of UCPs and facilitators, as described in this chapter, extend and support these findings by suggesting that more democratic, collaborative, and supportive social relations in LTC homes might provide UCPs as the primary care providers with the motivation and autonomy to strive toward practice excellence. UCPs need to be recognized for their contributions to resident care, involved in discussions about resident care, and actively solicited by all healthcare team members to contribute their practice opinions.

Another lesson to take away from the stories shared in this chapter is the importance of being clear about what we are asking of healthcare practitioners and what is required of them, both on an intellectual level and an emotional level as human beings, to implement best practices in the context of their work world. The care of older persons in LTC homes is complex, largely in relation to the challenges associated with dementia care specifically. There are gaps in the intellectual capacities of UCPs, by virtue of their minimal formal preparation that compromises their capacity to critically think through the best way to respond to difficult practice moments. However, in equal need of attention are the emotive capacities of UCPs required to sustain best practices to spite the stressors they face on a moment-by-moment basis. It would be difficult for any healthcare provider to demonstrate best practices when experiencing an overwhelming sense of frustration, resentment, fear, or burnout, regardless of the level of formal education they have. It is important to support UCPs in developing the emotional maturity to manage their feelings and cope in such a way that the feelings do not interfere with their capacity to reach their practice potentials. UCPs need to receive recognition from their leaders for their efforts to provide best practice, whatever the outcome. They need the right development and support opportunities to sustain their propensity for caring and maintain their composure in the face of the threat they experience from the behaviors of residents with ADRD.

This chapter presented the perspectives of UCPs and facilitators about evidence-based aged care. The views of LTC home administrators and registered nursing staff are still in need of investigation and would, very likely, contribute additional insight on how goals for better aged care practices can be realized. In light of the phenomenon of global aging, this research agenda is important on an international level. I have begun this by sharing views from the point-of-care in the Canadian context about the challenges facing us in LTC homes. My hope is to ultimately translate these views into strategies for facilitating excellence in the care received by older persons.

References

Alzheimer's Disease International (2009). *World Alzheimer Report 2009 Executive Summary*. London: Alzheimer's Disease International. Retrieved October 24, 2009, from http://www.alz.co.uk/research/files/WorldAlzheimerReport-ExecutiveSummary.pdf.

Bowers, B.J., Faan, S.E. & Jacobson, N. (2003). Turnover reinterpreted: CNAs talk about why they leave. *Journal of Gerontological Nursing*, 29, 36–43.

Caspar, S. & O'Rourke, N. (2008). The influence of care provider access to structural empowerment on individualized care in long-term care facilities. *The Journals of Gerontology. Series B, Psychological Sciences and Social Sciences*, 63B(4), S255–S265.

Chappell, N., Reid, R. & Gish, J.A. (2006). Staff-based measures of individualized care for persons with dementia in long-term care facilities. *Dementia: The International Journal of Social Research and Practice*, 6, 527–547.

Cohen-Mansfield, J. (2000). Nonpharmacological management of behavioural problems in persons with dementia: The TREA model. *Alzheimer Care Quarterly*, 1, 22–34.

Cohen-Mansfield, J. & Purpura-Gill, A. (2008). Practice style in the nursing home: Dimensions for assessment and quality improvement. *International Journal of Geriatric Psychiatry*, 23, 376–386.

Cready, C., Yeatts, D., Gosdin, M. & Potts, H. (2008). CNA empowerment: Effects on job performance and work attitudes. *Journal of Gerontological Nursing*, 34(3), 26–34.

Fläckman, B., Sørlie, V. & Kihlgren, M. (2008). Unmet expectations: Why nursing home staff leave care work. *International Journal of Older People Nursing*, 3, 55–62.

Janes, N., Sidani, S., Cott, C. & Rappolt, S. (2008). Figuring it out in the moment: A theory of unregulated care providers' knowledge utilization in dementia care settings. *Worldviews on Evidence Based Nursing*, 5(1), 13–24.

Janes, N., Fox, M., Lowe, M., McGilton, K. & Schindel-Martin, L. (2009). Facilitating best practice in aged care: Exploring influential factors through critical incident technique. *International Journal of Older People Nursing*, 4, 166–176.

Karlsson, I., Ekman, S. & Fagerberg, I. (2008). To both be like a captain and fellow worker of the caring team: The meaning of nurse assistants' expectations of registered nurses in Swedish residential care homes. *International Journal of Older People Nursing*, 3, 35–45.

Lau, W., Shyu, Y., Lin, L. & Yang, P. (2008). Institutionalized elders with dementia: Collaboration between family caregivers and nursing home staff in Taiwan. *Journal of Clinical Nursing*, 17, 482–490.

Lipe, S. & Beasley, S. (2004). *Critical Thinking in Nursing: A Cognitive Skills Workbook*. Philadelphia, PA: Lippincott Williams and Wilkins.

McCormack, B. (2004). Person-centeredness in gerontological nursing: An overview of the literature. *International Journal of Older People Nursing*, 13, 31–38.

McGilton, K. (2002). Enhancing relationships between care providers and residents in long-term care: Designing a model of care. *Journal of Gerontological Nursing*; 28(12), 13–20.

McPhaul, K.M. & Lipscomb, J.A. (2004). Workplace violence in health care: Recognized but not regulated. *Online Journal of Issues in Nursing*, 9(3), 6. Available at www.nursingworld.org/MainMenuCategories/ANA Marketplace/ANAPeriodicals/OJIN/TableofContents/Volume92004/No3Sept04/ViolenceinHealthCare.aspx.

Moise, P., Schwarzinger, M., Um, M. & the Dementia Experts' Group (2004). Dementia care in 9 OECD countries: A comparative analysis. *OECD Health Working Papers*. Available at http://www.oecd.org/LongAbstract/0,2546,en_2649_33929_33661492_119684_1_1_1,00.html.

OANHSS (1998). *Discussion Paper on the Registered Nurse in Long Term Care*. Woodbridge: Ontario Association of Non-profit Homes & Services for Seniors.

OCS Association (2009). Ministry of Health and Long Term Care Personal Support Worker Training Standards (1997). Retrieved November 16, 2009, from http://www.ocsa.on.ca/userfiles/PSW_Training_Standards.pdf.

OECD (2005). Ensuring quality long-term care for older people. *OECD Policy Brief*. Available at http://www.oecd.org/publications/policybriefs.

OECD (2007). Health data 2007: Statistics & indicators for 30 countries. Available at http://www.oecd.org.

Olson, D. & Zwygart-Stauffacher, M. (2008). The organizational quality frontier and essential role of the director of nursing. *Journal of Nursing Care Quality*, 23(1), 11–13.

Ontario Nurses Association (ONA) (2007). Submission on Bill 140—*Long-Term Care Homes Act, 2006* to the Standing Committee on Social Policy. Retrieved November 16, 2009, from http://www.ona.org/20070117ONANews.

Ontario Seniors' Secretariat (2007). A guide to programs and services for seniors in Ontario. Retrieved November 16, 2009, from http://www.culture.gov.on.ca/seniors/english/programs/seniorsguide/docs/SeniorsGuide.English.pdf.

Owen, T. (2008). Healthcare in care homes: A vision for improvement. *Journal of Community Nursing*, 22, 10–14.

Robinson, K.M. & Tappen, R.M. (2008). Policy recommendations on the prevention of violence in long-term care facilities. *Journal of Gerontological Nursing*, 34(3), 10–14.

Skovdahl, K., Kihlgren, A.L. & Kihlgren, M. (2003). Dementia and aggressiveness: Video recorded morning care from different care units. *Journal of Clinical Nursing*, 12(6), 888–898.

Teeri, S., Välimäki, M., Katajisto, J. & Leino-Kilpi, H. (2008). Maintenance of patients' integrity in long-term institutional care. *Nursing Ethics*, 15(4), 523–535.

Tellis-Nayak, V. (2007). A person-centered workplace: The foundation for person-centered caregiving in long-term care. *Journal of the American Medical Directors Association*, 8, 46–54.

WHO (2003). Ethical issues in long-term care. World Health Organization site. Online. Available at http://www.who.int/ethics/nfp_disabled/en/ (accessed June 13, 2009).

Chapter 10

Enabling context with policy

Gill Harvey

As other chapters in this book highlight, there are many factors in the practice context that can influence the uptake of evidence into clinical practice—relationships amongst team members, support and commitment from leadership, and the extent to which evaluation and reflection on practice is encouraged, to name just a few. But what about the wider policy context in which implementation takes place? Does this matter in terms of implementing evidence into practice at a clinical level? If so, how and why does it matter? This chapter will explore issues relating to the wider policy context of implementation, looking in particular at the relationships between policy and practice in relation to delivering evidence-based health care. Influences on decision making at a policy level will be discussed, drawing on specific examples to illustrate how the policy process can mediate the translation of evidence into practice, pushing some issues higher up the agenda and others lower down. Implications for planning implementing strategies at a clinical level that take account of the wider policy environment will be presented.

Introduction

Evidence-based health care is a high-level priority for governments across the world. Since the initial emergence of the evidence-based medicine movement (Sackett et al., 1996), the basic idea that decisions should be more systematically based on sound evidence of effectiveness has spread to other disciplines in health care, other areas of the public sector and to other levels of decision making. Subsequently, we see the term "evidence-based" used as a prefix to everything from nursing, physiotherapy, and dentistry to education, social work, and criminal justice, and more generally to management and policy.

Focusing specifically on health care, initial developments in evidence-based practice emerged from the clinical level, in response to widely recognized gaps between known evidence of best practice and what was actually happening in terms of the delivery of clinical care. For example, some studies (Grol, 2001; Schuster et al., 1998) have suggested that 30–40% of patients do not receive care complying with current scientific evidence. Responding to these concerns, early developments focused on the synthesis of research evidence in the form of systematic reviews, establishing review groups to coordinate and undertake this work, for example, through the Cochrane Collaboration, and teaching clinicians skills in accessing and critically appraising research evidence. Over time, these initiatives became supported by further developments at a policy level, such as the establishment of national bodies to collate, synthesize, and publish evidence, typically in the form of clinical guidelines and technology appraisals, for example, relating to the treatment of people with particular conditions, or for specific clinical and pharmaceutical interventions (Lewis, 2001; Miller & Petrie, 2000; Rawlins, 1999). National demonstration projects to develop and disseminate models and exemplars for translating research into practice were established (Dopson et al., 2001; Wallin et al., 2000), and research programs were funded to investigate and increase understanding about the most effective methods and processes for getting research into practice (AHRQ, 2001; Hanney et al., 2003).

However, despite the heavy investment in evidence-based health care at both policy and practice levels, translating research in to health care decision making and practice remains a considerable challenge. For example, the Institute of Medicine in the USA established a Clinical Research Roundtable to address the issues facing the national research enterprise and concluded that failure to translate new knowledge into clinical practice and health care decision making was one of the two major barriers preventing human benefit from the advances in biomedical sciences (Sung et al., 2003). Similarly in the UK, the Cooksey Report on UK health research funding (HM Treasury, 2006) identified the failure to implement new technologies and approaches into health care practice as the "second translation gap." Despite establishing a national body, the

National Institute for Health and Clinical Excellence (NICE), in England and Wales to undertake technology appraisals and produce clinical guidelines for the National Health Service (NHS), evaluations of the extent and pattern of implementation of guidance issued by NICE demonstrate highly variable levels of uptake, ranging from no change to significant changes in practice in line with the guidance (Raftery, 2006; Sheldon et al., 2004).

Understanding the reasons why such gaps in knowledge translation exist has led to closer examination of the processes involved in disseminating and implementing evidence into practice. Early models of evidence-based practice, which assumed a rational, linear approach to implementation (e.g., Haines & Jones, 1994) have been criticized as oversimplistic and failing to recognize the complex, messy world of changing clinical practice (Kitson et al., 1998; Nutley et al., 2007). One factor that emerges strongly as an influence on the uptake of evidence in clinical practice is the context, or environment, in which practice takes place (Cummings et al., 2007; Dopson & Fitzgerald, 2005; McCormack et al., 2002; Rycroft-Malone et al., 2002). As the other chapters in this book illustrate, context itself is a multilayered and multidimensional concept, incorporating various elements of the immediate organizational environment. However, health care organizations rarely exist in isolation—that is to say, they are typically part of a wider public sector health service or a group of independent providers. This imposes another layer of context that can influence attempts to implement evidence into practice, namely, the policy context. In the case of publicly funded health systems, this policy context is shaped by government, although decision making may take place at various levels of national, regional and local policy making. In privately funded health systems, the policy context will be shaped by a combination of government policy and company-level strategy and policy.

To what extent does this wider policy context really matter in terms of implementing evidence into clinical practice? How does the policy process influence evidence-based decision making at a clinical level? And how important is it to be aware of and take into account the policy context when planning implementation strategies at a local level? This chapter will attempt to answer some of these questions, firstly by examining the processes involved in policy making and the part that research evidence plays in that process. The relationship between policy and practice will then be discussed, including strategies for bridging the gap between the two groups and creating a policy context that enhances and enables evidence-based practice at a clinical level.

Evidence and policy making

As highlighted in the introduction, in many ways policy makers have embraced the evidence-based health care agenda, for example, through expressing a commitment to closing the evidence–practice gap and establishing a supporting infrastructure to further the development of evidence-based practice. Indeed, the growth of the evidence-based health care movement prompted increasing calls for similar evidence-based approaches to be applied to the processes of decision making at the managerial and policy levels of health care (Walshe & Rundall, 2001). We could perhaps assume from this, therefore, that with policy makers, managers and health care managers all committed to an evidence-based approach, there should exist a highly supportive context for delivering evidence-based health care to patients and the public. However, like most things, the reality of the situation is less straightforward than it perhaps sounds on paper. As Ray Pawson (2006, p. viii) eloquently puts it when considering the term "evidence-based policy":

> The problem with the term, and it is quite a big one, is that there is no such thing as evidence-based policy. Evidence is the six stone weakling of the policy world.

Does this mean that the commitment to an evidence-based approach is merely rhetoric and not followed through in practice? In attempting to understand this, it is helpful to take a step backward and examine what happens when policy is made, key influences on the policy process and the place of evidence amongst those influences.

The policy-making process

Policy can be defined as "a position taken on an issue by an organization or individual in a position of power" (Baggott, 2007, p. 2). According to Colebatch (2002), policy comprises three central elements:

(1) It is concerned with order, implying a systematic and consistent approach.
(2) It is legitimized by the authority of individuals, offices, or organizations.
(3) It is underpinned by various bodies of expertise, including theories and findings relating to problems and ways these might be resolved.

> **Box 10.1 Some definitions of health policy**
>
> Health policy is assumed to embrace courses of action (and inaction) that affect the set of institutions, organizations, services and funding arrangements of the health system. It includes policy made in the public sector (by government) as well as policies in the private sector
>
> (Buse et al., 2005, p. 6)
>
> Those courses of action proposed or taken by a government that impact on the financing and/or provision of health services
>
> (Blank & Burau, 2004, p. 16)
>
> Health policy is about process and power . . . it is concerned with who influences whom in the making of policy, and how that happens
>
> (Walt, 1994, p. 1)

Drawing on these principles, a number of definitions of health policy have been proposed (see Box 10.1). Emerging from these definitions are several core aspects of health policy, concerning its role in driving the purpose and direction of health care provision and the influence of power within these processes. As Buse et al. (2005, p. 1) point out:

> Who makes and implements policy decisions (those with power) and how decisions are made (process) largely determine the content of health policy and, thereby, ultimately, people's health.

Debates about how the policy-making process works share something in common with the differing views on how to implement evidence-based health care, with examples ranging from rational, linear models of policy making (e.g., Hogwood & Gunn, 1984; Simon, 1945) to more multifaceted, iterative frameworks to explain the process (e.g., Buse et al., 2005; Walt & Gilson, 1994; Weiss, 1999). Buse et al. (2005), drawing on the work of Walt and Gilson (1994), suggest a policy triangle, which takes account of the content, context, processes, and actors involved in the policy process and the interrelationships between them (see Figure 10.1). Walt and Gilson's original view was that too often discussions about health policy focused simply on the content of the policy, with little consideration of the people (actors) involved, the processes contingent on developing and implementing change, and the context within which

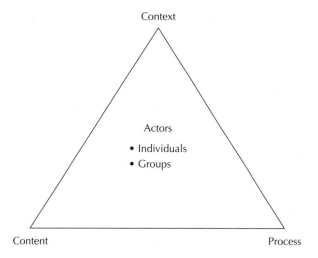

Figure 10.1 The policy analysis triangle.
Source: Walt and Gilson (1994). Reprinted with permission from *Healthy Policy and Planning*.

policy is developed. The result of this, they suggested, was a poor understanding of why policy changes sometimes failed to achieve the desired impact:

> Focus on policy content diverts attention from understanding the processes which explain why desired policy outcomes fail to emerge.

> (Walt & Gilson, 1994, p. 353)

Actors are at the center of the health framework proposed by Walt and Gilson (1994). These actors may be individuals, groups, or organizations, who exercise power in an attempt to try and influence the policy process. Examples in health care could include professional organizations, consumers and patients, patient representative groups, government departments or international bodies such as the World Health Organization or the European Union (EU). The extent to which actors can successfully influence policy will depend partly on the level of power they can exercise, which in turn relates to a range of factors including resources, availability of knowledge, authority, and the organizational structures to which they are aligned (Buse et al., 2005).

Contextual factors that can influence policy have been described as situational, structural, cultural, and international (Leichter, 1979). Situational factors are transient or unpredictable events that can impact on health policy, for example, a crisis event such as war or a natural disaster, or the emergence of a new disease, as was the case with HIV and AIDS. Structural factors are the more permanent features and include the political system, demographic characteristics of the population, the economic state, level of wealth, and so on. Cultural factors encompass a range of attitudes, values, and beliefs that may be influenced, amongst other things, by religious views and the level of democracy that exists. International factors refer to issues where cooperation across national boundaries may be required, for example, to tackle particular diseases or issues on a more global scale, such as when a major flu pandemic arises, or the international patient safety movement.

The policy process is concerned with the way in which policies are devised, developed, negotiated, implemented, and evaluated. Whilst this process is often presented as a staged approach, moving from problem identification to policy formulation, implementation, and evaluation (Hogwood & Gunn, 1984), as the earlier discussion highlights, interpretations of the process as a purely rational, linear one have largely been rejected in favor of more interactive, dynamic approaches, sometimes referred to as incremental approaches to policy making, or what Lindblom (1959) described as the "science of muddling through."

Key to understanding this more multifaceted view of policy is taking account of the complex interrelationships between the different elements involved, rather than viewing each in isolation. As Buse et al. (2005, p. 9) point out:

> In reality, actors are influenced (as individuals or members of groups or organizations) by the context within which they live and work; context is affected by many factors such as instability or ideology, by history and culture; and the process of policy making – how issues get on policy agendas, and how they fare once there – is affected by actors, their position in power structures, their own values and expectations. And the content of policy reflects some or all of these dimensions.

Weiss (1999) proposed that the four elements of interests, ideology, information, and institutions are at play in shaping the context within which policy making takes place. In her analysis, interests are largely the self-interests of those engaged in the policy process, and could be both political and personal. Ideology refers to the beliefs, morals, political orientations, and ethical values that guide the decision making and actions of policy makers. Information includes the wide range of knowledge and ideas that policy makers draw on to make sense of current issues and plan policy solutions (of which evidence may be just one component), whilst institutions are the organizations within which policy makers act. These institutions come with their own culture and history, which in turn can exert influence on the other elements of interests, ideologies, and information.

The place of evidence in the policy process

As this brief overview of health policy and the policy process illustrates, there is a complex set of influences at work. It is perhaps not surprising therefore, that evidence does not automatically or easily translate into new policy decisions or frameworks. Indeed, the similarities between the complexities of implementing evidence-based practice and evidence-based policy are in many ways striking. So what, if any, part can evidence play in the process of making policy decisions and are there ways in which the policy context can be made more supportive of evidence-based clinical practice?

In considering the first issue, the place of evidence in policy making, it is useful first to think about the different ways in which evidence might be used in decision making. Early attempts to promote and achieve evidence-based practice often focused on the direct or so-called instrumental, use of evidence in practice. However, many studies have demonstrated that evidence rarely gets used in such a direct or straightforward way, sometimes because the evidence is not definitive, and even when it is, because of the complex processes of negotiation and contestation at the level of implementation (e.g., Dopson & Fitzgerald, 2005; Nutley et al., 2007). Instead, evidence often finds its way into decision making, at both the practice and policy level, through more indirect routes, for example, by raising awareness or challenging existing ways of thinking. This type of evidence use is often described as conceptual and involves changing perceptions, rather than bringing about immediate changes to policy or practice (Nutley et al., 2007).

Studies into the use of research evidence by policy makers suggest that they are more likely to use evidence in a conceptual, as opposed to instrumental, way. For example, a review by Innvaer and colleagues (2002) of health policy makers' use of research showed rates of conceptual use up to 20% higher than instrumental use. Indeed, many policy makers report limited direct application of research evidence because of its perceived lack of relevance, or the material being too detailed, dense, or technical (Sorian & Baugh, 2002).

As Nutley et al. (2007, p. 37) point out, evidence may also be used in strategic or tactical ways:

> It can be used as an instrument of persuasion, to support an existing political stance or to challenge the positions of others. It can also be deployed to legitimate a decision or course of action.

Or, as Pawson (2006, p. viii) notes when reflecting on the relatively weak position of evidence in the policy-making process, perhaps "policy-based evidence" is a more accurate term to use when thinking about how evidence is really used within the policy process. Empirical findings from research suggest that strategic use of evidence is in fact more prevalent than instrumental use amongst policy makers (Innvaer et al., 2002).

Consequently, it appears unrealistic, or at least unlikely, to expect policy makers to receive and apply evidence in a purely instrumental way. Alongside the different ways in which evidence can be used, it is also important to take account of what concerns policy makers in relation to the quality of health care. Typically, policy makers work with broad definitions of quality, reflecting a range of dimensions, such as the Institute of Medicine's definition of quality in terms of the safety, effectiveness, patient-centeredness, timeliness, efficiency, and equity of health care (Institute of Medicine, 2001). This is in contrast to the traditional focus of the evidence-based health care movement which has, to a large extent, been concerned with questions of effectiveness. So, for example, the research evidence may indicate the best way to manage or treat a particular condition, but at a policy level, questions of optimal effectiveness have to be set alongside considerations of efficiency, equity, appropriateness, and acceptability, particularly within the resource constraints of the public sector environment.

From his earlier ideas of rational policy making (Simon, 1945), Simon subsequently put forward the notion of "bounded rationality," arguing that people were typically unable to deal with complex problems in a purely objective way (Simon, 1957). From this premise, Simon (1957) suggested that instead of aiming for optimal outcomes, most policy makers would opt for a good enough solution, a concept referred to as satisficing. In line with this school of thinking, it has been argued that policy makers have a tendency to make pragmatic decisions, focused on short-term solutions (Lomas, 1997). Add to this that many policy decisions are concerned with questions of quality and service provision at the population level, whereas discussions on evidence-based practice at the clinical level may be more individually focused, and the potential for divergent or conflicting priorities becomes clear (McInnes et al., 2001).

From policy to practice

Having considered some of the influences on health policy and the different ways in which evidence might be used in the policy process, the next set of questions to think about is to what extent the prevailing policy environment influences the implementation of evidence-based practice at a clinical level. From the preceding discussion, it should be clear that the multifaceted practice environment itself sits within a complex, multilayered policy environment, which could potentially act to enhance or limit the chances of successfully implementing evidence into practice. Whilst clinically the evidence may support a particular course of action, whether and how this evidence gets implemented into practice will depend on a range of organizational and policy-level influences, including current priorities, resource availability, the role of interest groups and the media, societal values and beliefs, to name just a view.

This can be illustrated by analyzing the case of fertility treatment in the National Health Service (NHS) in England (see Box 10.2). This example suggests that the guideline had a limited, and at best variable, impact on the provision of in vitro fertilization to couples experiencing fertility problems. Consider some of the factors within the external policy environment (at both a national and local level) that you think might have influenced the level of uptake of this evidence in practice (see Box 10.3).

> **Box 10.2 The case of fertility treatment in the National Health Service in England**
>
> In response to concerns about the inequity of access to treatment for infertility in the NHS, the Department of Health (national policy level) commissioned the National Institute for Health and Clinical Excellence (NICE) to produce a set of national clinical guidelines on assessment and treatment for people with fertility problems. These guidelines were published in 2004 (NICE, 2004) and disseminated with accompanying implementation and audit guidance and projected budget implications to regional- and local-level policy makers (strategic health authorities and primary care commissioners). Over 12 months after issuing the guidelines, two follow-up surveys were conducted amongst fertility experts and primary care trust (PCT) commissioning managers to assess the impact of the guideline (NICE, 2005a,b).
>
> In the original guideline, one of the seven key priorities for implementation concerned the number of cycles of in vitro fertilization (IVF) to be provided:
>
> > Couples in which the woman is aged 23–39 years at the time of treatment and who have identified cause for their fertility problems (such as azoospermia or bilateral tubal occlusion) or who have infertility of at least 5 years' duration should be offered up to three stimulated cycles of IVF treatment.
> >
> > (NICE, 2005a, p. 4)
>
> The subsequent follow-up survey examined the extent to which this priority had been met. In the majority of PCTs (63.5%), couples who met the eligibility criteria for IVF were offered just one cycle of treatment (NICE, 2005a). No PCTs were offering three cycles of IVF. From the survey of fertility experts, 64.3% reported that the guideline had made no difference to the provision of IVF (NICE, 2005b).

Taking account of policy in implementation strategies

If we accept, as this chapter has attempted to put forward, that the prevailing policy environment does exert some influence over the practice environment in which evidence-based decisions are made, what do we need to think about when planning strategies for evidence-based practice at a clinical level? How can we assess the extent to which the external policy environment will influence the changes we want to introduce? What will be the likely direction of

> **Box 10.3 Reflections on the policy environment and its influence on the uptake of evidence on fertility treatment in practice**
>
> - What factors in the external policy environment might have influenced the level of uptake of evidence?
> - Who do you think the key actors might have been?
> - What contextual factors might have been at play (e.g., structural, situational, and cultural?)
> - Think about a similar example of fertility treatment within your own health setting. Would you expect the response to this guideline to be similar or different? Why?
> - Can you think of other guideline topics where the uptake in practice has been more successful? What are the reasons for this? How influential was the wider policy environment?

this influence—supportive or restrictive? And what actions could we take to try and build a more enabling policy environment that supports the implementation of evidence into practice?

It is perhaps useful at this point to recap on some of the key points that have emerged from the discussion of health policy in relation to evidence based practice so far:

(1) Health policy making is a complex activity, influenced by the actors involved, the context in which it takes place and the nature of the policy-making process.

(2) The policy context comprises a number of different structural, situational, and cultural factors and can be seen to be shaped by a combination of interests, ideology, information, and institutions.

(3) Rational models of the policy process fail to represent the reality of what happens; in practice, the policy process is typically iterative and incremental in nature.

(4) Policy makers are more likely to use research evidence in conceptual and strategic ways, as opposed to the more direct or instrumental application of evidence.

(5) Policy makers are concerned with a broad range of issues pertaining to quality, of which the effectiveness of care is just one element.

(6) These broader dimensions of quality, for example, efficiency, acceptability, timeliness, and equity, can exert a powerful influence when decisions about implementing evidence into practice are taken at a local level.

(7) Policy makers often aim for pragmatic, good enough solutions in relation to complex problems and competing priorities.
(8) Policy decisions are typically taken at the population level, as opposed to the care of individual patients.

How might this help when thinking about evidence-based change that is being planned at a clinical level? Harrison (2001) cited by Buse et al. (2005, p. 160) suggests at least seven conditions that, hypothetically, need to be met for the ideal or perfect implementation of research evidence in clinical practice:

(1) the existence of comprehensive, authoritative statements based on rigorous reviews of research evidence
(2) the ability of such statements to provide a direct guide to decision making in specific clinical circumstances
(3) knowledge of such statements by all relevant actors
(4) adequate resources to act upon the authoritative evidence
(5) sufficient incentive to apply the evidence
(6) absence of substantial disincentives to apply the evidence
(7) an implementation chain sufficiently short to ensure a good likelihood of compliance with the implications of the evidence.

In one sense, these conditions could comprise the perfect situation in which direct, instrumental application of evidence could occur. However, the likelihood of such a set of conditions existing in the real world of clinical practice seems extremely rare. As conceptual models such as the Promoting Action on Research Implementation in Health Services (PARIHS) framework highlight, evidence is a contested and multifaceted concept, comprising research evidence, alongside clinical and patient experience and local information (Rycroft-Malone et al., 2004). Unless these different components of evidence are aligned, then the existence of strong evidence to drive implementation is unlikely. Rather, evidence is likely to be contested, disputed, and negotiated because of competing perceptions, values, and interests. Add to this the complex nature of the practice context (McCormack et al., 2002) and the importance of how the implementation process itself is facilitated (Harvey et al., 2002) and it is probably fair to conclude that an ideal set of conditions for the straightforward or relatively easy translation of research evidence into practice is just that—an ideal vision.

If instead, we accept that the process of implementing evidence into practice is complex, multifaceted, and context dependent, so it becomes increasingly likely that the policy environment has a part to play in shaping the context for implementation and ultimately influencing the success or otherwise of the implementation effort. As a first step in assessing the policy environment in which implementation is taking place, it is useful to think about the evidence-based practice changes to be introduced and where these sit in relation to policy-related issues (see Box 10.4). The more your planned changes are aligned with strategic priorities, are clearly based on sound baseline data, and are strongly supported (at the level of patients, colleagues, managers, and wider stakeholders), the greater the likelihood of successful implementation.

However, assuming you undertake a quick analysis of the wider environment and realize that the changes you want to introduce are not strongly in line with current priorities and indeed may have to compete with these strategic priorities for support and resources, what then? Are there things you could do to build a stronger case for change and create a more supportive context for implementation? In exploring these questions, it is helpful to look at some of the literature on bridging the gaps between policy, research and practice, and strategies that can be employed to support this.

Box 10.4 Assessing the policy environment for implementing evidence-based practice

- To what extent are your planned changes aligned with national, regional, or local policy priorities?
- What information or data (e.g., audit data, patient stories, and feedback from carers) have you collated to support the need for change?
- How does this information match with research evidence on the same subject?
- What resources (financial, time, etc.) will you need to support implementation? How you are planning to secure these?
- What support will you need from policy makers at an organizational level or beyond to implement the changes that you have planned?
- Are there national or local policy documents that you could draw on to support your case?

Bridging the gaps between practice, policy, and research

As we have already discovered, policy making is rarely a rational process. Therefore securing policy-level support for proposed evidence-based changes in practice is not simply a case of presenting strong, robust research evidence to policy makers. If policy makers are more likely to make use of research evidence in conceptual and strategic ways, this is important to bear in mind when considering strategies for securing support.

One useful framework that has been put forward to explain the relationship between research and policy is Crewe and Young's context-evidence-links model (Crewe & Young, 2002). Underpinned by a belief that policy making is "structured by a complex interplay between political interests, competing discourses and the agency of multiple actors" (Crewe & Young, 2002, p. 3), the framework draws on and aims to integrate a wide range of underlying theories to examine the way in which the nature of the research, the context, and linkages between key players shape whether and how research is used in the process of policy making (Nutley et al., 2007). The uptake of research evidence in policy is seen as a function of the interaction between evidence, context, and links (see Table 10.1). In many ways, this echoes the basic proposition of the PARIHS framework, which suggests that the uptake of research evidence in practice is a function of the relationship between evidence, context, and facilitation (or the way in which the process of implementation is facilitated) (Kitson et al., 1998).

This is a useful point of comparison, because it serves to highlight the similarities between contextual influences on implementation at the practice and policy level. It is, however, important to remember that the policy environment is likely to include a broader range of influences on decision making, not least of which are political in nature, and a need to satisfy a wide range of requirements at the population level. The net result of this may be that issues that seem to be of paramount importance at the clinical level might seem less significant or urgent at the policy level because of competing interests, different priorities, a short-term agenda, and so on. Nonetheless, it is useful to note the similar direction of travel in terms of frameworks for evidence-based practice and evidence-based (or evidence-informed) policy, as this suggests that strategies for creating a supportive context at the clinical, organizational level could

Table 10.1 The context-evidence-links model of the research–policy relationship

Context	Evidence	Links
Political and institutional structures and the distribution of power within these	Credibility of research	Use of research will be greater where researchers and policy makers have closer links
Interests and roles of policy makers and researchers	Methods of communication	Importance of "chains of legitimacy"
Organizational cultures and pressures within which policy makers and researchers act	Quality of research, its source, and the way it is packaged	Role of policy networks and policy entrepreneurs in integrating research and policy
	Interactions between researchers and policy makers	
	Influence of policy makers' preexisting knowledge, values, and experience	

Source: Informed by Crewe and Young (2002).

be usefully transferred to the wider policy context—albeit with some adjustments, amendments, and fine-tuning.

Of particular relevance in Crewe and Young's evidence-context-links framework is the links dimension. This highlights the importance of close collaboration and an engaged relationship between researchers and policy makers, rather than existing as two distinct groups. Different ways of achieving this more engaged approach include the use of policy networks or the developing linkage and exchange models, with an explicit role for knowledge purveyors bridging the gap between research and policy (Lomas, 2000; Nutley et al., 2007).

Returning to the issue of the policy–practice relationship and ways of influencing policy to create a more conducive environment, the ideas around linkage hold some important messages in terms of building engagement and dialogue with key stakeholders and decision makers at various levels of the policy-making process. In line with the various multidimensional, interactive models of decision making, such dialogue needs to involve a two-way process of communication that is iterative and flexible. At a local level, this means thinking about who are the key stakeholders that need to be engaged at the outset of the planned change or implementation project, rather than half way down the line or when things are not going as planned. And the engagement has to be just that, a process of consulting with and gaining feedback from stakeholders (which will comprise a wider group, but include policy makers) to shape, refine, and evaluate the implementation plan as it progresses. This is unlikely to be a simple or straightforward process and will undoubtedly require negotiation and compromise. However, the investment up front to secure engagement and support should reap dividends as implementation progresses, including the subsequent stages of sustaining and spreading new practice.

Summary

This chapter has attempted to demonstrate the influence of policy in shaping the context within which evidence-based practice is delivered at a clinical level. Not dissimilar to the practice context, the policy context is seen to influence and be influenced by a range of interrelated factors linked to individual and organizational characteristics, alongside issues of power and politics. Put simply, policy represents an additional, outer layer of the context in which evidence-based practice occurs. As such, awareness and consideration of this broader policy context and its likely influence on the successful implementation of evidence at a clinical level is essential, as are strategies for creating dialogue and engagement with policy makers to build an optimal environment for implementation.

References

Agency for Health Research and Quality (AHRQ) (2001). *Translating Research into Practice II (TRIP II)*. Washington DC: AHRQ.

Baggott, R. (2007). *Understanding Health Policy*. Bristol: The Policy Press.

Blank, R. & Burau, V. (2004). *Comparative Health Policy*. Basingstoke: Palgrave Macmillan.

Buse, K., Mays, N. & Watt, G. (2005). *Making Health Policy*. Maidenhead: Open University Press.

Colebatch, H. (2002). *Policy*, 2nd ed. Buckingham: Open University Press.

Crewe, E. & Young, J. (2002). *Bridging Research and Policy: Context, Evidence and Links*. London: Overseas Development Institute.

Cummings, G.G., Estabrooks, C.A., Midozi, W.K., Wallin, L. & Hayduk, L. (2007). Influence of organisational characteristics and context on research utilisation. *Nursing Research*, 56(4S), S24–S39.

Dopson, S. & Fitzgerald, L. (2005). *Knowledge to Action? Evidence-based Healthcare in Context*. Oxford: Oxford University Press.

Dopson, S., Locock, L., Chamber, D. & Gabbay, J. (2001). Implementation of evidence-based medicine: Evaluation of the Promoting Action on Clinical Effectiveness Programme. *Journal of Health Services Research and Policy*, 6(1), 23–31.

Grol, R. (2001). Successes and failures in the implementation of evidence-based guidelines for clinical practice. *Medical Care*, 39(8 Suppl. II), 46–54.

Haines, A. & Jones, R. (1994). Implementing findings of research. *British Medical Journal*, 308, 1488–1492.

Hanney, S., Soper, B. & Buxton, M. (2003). *Evaluation of the NHS R&D Implementation Methods Programme*. London: Health Economics Research Group, Brunel University.

Harvey, G., Loftus-Hills, A., Rycroft-Malone, J. et al. (2002). Getting evidence into practice: The role and function of facilitation. *Journal of Advanced Nursing*, 37(6), 577–588.

HM Treasury (2006). *A Review of UK Health Research Funding*: Sir David Cooksey. London: HM Treasury. Available at http://www.hm-treasury. gov.uk/d/pbr06_cooksey_final_report_636.pdf.

Hogwood, B. & Gunn, L. (1984). *Policy Analysis for the Real World*. Oxford: Oxford University Press.

Innvaer, S., Vist, G., Trommald, M. & Oxman, A.D. (2002). Health policy-makers' perceptions of their use of evidence: A systematic review. *Journal of Health Services Research and Policy*, 17(4), 239–244.

Institute of Medicine, Committee on Quality Health Care in America (2001). *Crossing the Quality Chasm*. Washington DC: Institute of Medicine.

Kitson, A., Harvey G. & McCormack, B. (1998). Enabling the implementation of evidence based practice: A conceptual framework. *Quality in Health Care*, 7(3), 149–159.

Leichter, H. (1979). *A Comparative Approach to Policy Analysis: Health Care Policy in Four Nations*. Cambridge: Cambridge University Press.

Lewis, D. (2001). National guideline clearing house: Extensive resource underused. *Managed Care*, 10(6), 41–42.

Lindblom, C. (1959). The science of muddling through. *Public Administration Review*, 19(2), 78–88.

Lomas, J. (1997), Reluctant rationers: Public input into health care priorities. *Journal of Health Services Research and Policy*, 2, 103–111.

Lomas, J. (2000). Using "linkage and exchange" to move research into policy at a Canadian foundation. *Health Affairs*, 19(3), 236–240.

McCormack, B., Kitson, A., Harvey, G., Rycroft-Malone, J., Titchen, A. & Seers, K. (2002). Getting evidence into practice: The meaning of context. *Journal of Advanced Nursing*, 38(1), 94–104.

McInnes, E., Harvey, G., Duff, L., Fennessy, G., Seers, K. & Clark, E. (2001). Implementing evidence-based practice in clinical situations. *Nursing Standard*, 15(41), 40–44.

Miller, J. & Petrie, J. (2000). Development of practice guidelines. *Lancet*, 355, 82–83.

National Institute for Health and Clinical Excellence (NICE) (2004). *Fertility: Assessment and Treatment for People with Fertility Problems*. London: RCOG Press.

National Institute for Health and Clinical Excellence (NICE) (2005a). *A Survey Measuring the Impact of NICE Guideline 11: Fertility: Assessment and Treatment for People with Fertility Problems. Survey One: PCT Commissioning Managers*. London: NICE.

National Institute for Health and Clinical Excellence (NICE) (2005b). *A Survey Measuring the Impact of NICE Guideline 11: Fertility: Assessment and Treatment for People with Fertility Problems. Survey Two: Fertility Experts*. London: NICE.

Nutley, S.M., Walter, I. & Davies, H.T.O. (2007). *Using Evidence: How Research Can Inform Public Services*. Bristol: The Policy Press.

Pawson, R. (2006). *Evidence-based Policy: A Realist Perspective*. London: Sage.

Raftery, J. (2006). Review of NICE's recommendations 1999–2005. *British Medical Journal*, 332, 1266–1268.

Rawlins, M. (1999). In pursuit of quality: The National Institute for Clinical Excellence. *Lancet*, 353, 1079–1082.

Rycroft-Malone, J., Kitson, A., Harvey, G. et al. (2002). Ingredients for change: Revisiting a conceptual framework. *Quality and Safety in Healthcare*, 11(2), 174–180.

Rycroft-Malone, J., Seers, K., Titchen, A., Harvey, G., Kitson, A. & McCormack, B. (2004). What counts as evidence in evidence-based practice? *Journal of Advanced Nursing*, 47(1), 81–90.

Sackett, D.L., Rosenberg, J.A. & Gray, R.B. (1996). Evidence based medicine: What it is and what it isn't. *British Medical Journal*, 312, 71–72.

Schuster, M., McGlynn, E. & Brook, R.H. (1998). How good is the quality of health care in the United States? *The Milbank Quarterly*, 76, 517–563.

Sheldon, T.A., Cullum, N., Dawson, D. et al. (2004). What's the evidence that NICE guidance has been implemented? Results from a national evaluation using time series analysis, audit of patients' notes, and interviews. *British Medical Journal*, 329(7473), 999.

Simon, H. (1945). *Administrative Behaviour*. Glencoe: Free Press.

Simon, H. (1957). *Models of Man*. New York: John Wiley and Sons.

Sorian, R. & Baugh, T. (2002). Power of information: Closing the gap between research and policy. *Health Affairs*, 21(2), 246–273.

Sung, N.S., Crowley, W.F., Genel, M. et al. (2003). Central challenges facing the national clinical research enterprise. *Journal of the American Medical Association*, 289, 1278–1287.

Wallin, L., Bostrom, A.M., Harvey, G., Wikbald, K. & Ewald, U. (2000). National guidelines for Swedish neonatal care: Evaluation of clinical application. *International Journal for Quality in Health Care*, 12(6), 465–474.

Walshe, K. & Rundall, T. (2001). Evidence based management: From theory to practice in healthcare. *The Milbank Quarterly*, 79(3), 429–457.

Walt, G. (1994). *Health Policy: An Introduction to Process and Power*. London: Zed Books.

Walt, G. & Gilson, L. (1994). Reforming the health sector in developing countries: The central role of policy analysis. *Health Policy and Planning*, 9, 353–370.

Weiss, C.H. (1999). The interface between evaluation and public policy. *Evaluation*, 5(4), 468–486.

Chapter 11

Context in context

Bridie Kent and Brendan McCormack

Introduction

This chapter, being the final one of this book, will synthesize the contextual factors for evidence-based practice that have been illustrated and expanded upon in the preceding chapters. The authors have captured the key contextual influences that impact upon evidence translation in various practice settings, ranging from primary care to the acute care environments and provided some excellent examples as illustrations. In isolation, each chapter portrays contextual factors that pose particular challenges to the successful translation of evidence into practice in specific settings. The examples given serve to provide readers with strategies, approaches, and, at the very least, ideas that have been shown to result in some form of evidence translation and practice change. However, when the chapters are taken together, they provide a very powerful toolkit of change strategies and help to emphasize those that are more effective at achieving change than others. In Chapter 2 we introduced McCormack et al.'s (2002) synthesis of context. These chapters move this work forward and set the scene for another systematic review, or possibly realist synthesis, to rigorously evaluate the strength of influence of the varying factors identified in this and other work. At the very least, this body of work begins to tell us more about the positive attributes of context that, when present, go towards providing the conditions for evidence to be used and for practice to be more effective. However, it is also clear that these attributes don't "just happen" but instead, they are dependent on a variety of conditions to be in place in order for them to exist—we refer to these as antecedents. In this chapter we will draw upon the previous chapters of this book and also discussions arising from the "Knowledge Utilization Colloquium"[1] which met in Wales in July 2009 (KU09).

Attributes of context

The chapters in this book clearly illustrate and reinforce the assertions of McCormack and colleagues (McCormack & Wright, 2009; McCormack et al., 2002) that there are a range of attributes that impact on context and the extent to which these play a part on the impact of evidence translation is determined by the setting itself. Some attributes could be described as being "hard" in nature and appear to be more easily visualized, for example structural boundaries, physical and environmental factors, and economic influences. These attributes are all evident to varying degrees in the chapters of this book. Structural and physical factors were more commonly identified in each of the different settings than economic influences but that is not to diminish its importance but instead may reflect an aspect of knowledge translation work that is as yet poorly developed. Economic and political factors affect all settings where healthcare takes place and directly or indirectly influences knowledge translation. Take for example the implementation of falls evidence in acute care settings. In 2008, a falls prevention best practice guideline was revised (Gray-Micelli, 2008) and yet across the world, falls continue to be a significant cause of adverse events and patient harm. Falls prevalence data are used, in many jurisdictions, as key quality indicators and programs such as Magnet Recognition™ and Transforming Care at the Bedside™ include such data as measures of performance and success. However, the implementation of falls prevention evidence is affected by economic factors. Not all countries can access the relevant evidence or be able to afford new technologies such as falls alarms that can help to alert staff immediately to a person who has fallen, thus limiting the damage caused by the fall. However, not all interventions for falls prevention are costly as illustrated in a practice improvement initiative by Murphy et al. (2008). They introduced interventions that included an awareness

---

[1] The Knowledge Utilization (KU) Colloquium is an international group of experts in the field of knowledge utilization and translation. The purpose of the KU group is to move the science of knowledge utilization forward in a focused and strategic way, leading to concrete outputs that extend our conceptual and theoretical development, and ultimately practice in knowledge utilization. The KU group meets annually and an archive of the work of the group can be found at http://www.kusp.ualberta.ca/KU0Xarchive.cfm.

raising campaign, "falls tool boxes," education of staff and family, and implementation of a structured hourly patient rounds schedule. Hourly patient rounding has also found success in the USA as reported on the AHRQ web site (http://www.innovations.ahrq.gov/content.aspx?id=2504) and, in ongoing research that is taking place in two acute care units in Melbourne, Australia. Changes to models of care delivery are resulting in significant reductions in falls (for more information on this project contact Bridie Kent).

Trying to introduce national guidelines is not without their associated problems. In a recent paper in *Worldviews on Evidence-Based Nursing*, blood transfusion practices were used to illustrate the difficulties that arise when new policy or a new guideline is introduced at a macro-level (Kent et al., 2009). Studies of blood transfusion practices resulted in the introduction of a national clinical practice guideline to enhance the safety around the administration of blood in the UK (British Committee for Standards in Haematology et al., 1999). In order to embed these standards into practice, changes needed to be made to ways of learning local and regional policies and ultimately changes in behavior. However, an audit of practice (Taylor et al., 2008) revealed that, in 2005, which was 6 years after the guidelines were first introduced, 6% of patients receiving a transfusion were found to have no form of patient identification (wristband or equivalent), and 13% had no transfusion-related observations recorded. These are essential aspects of patient safety and noncompliance places patients at risk. The reasons why practitioners have not embedded the activities identified above into their practice were not included in the audit; however, these may reflect the "soft" aspects of context such as having clarity of beliefs and values in a team, using learning as an integral component of clinical effectiveness, ensuring practitioners are clear about their responsibility for accountability and developing interprofessional relationships that are energy enhancing. Thus we can see that context is multilayered, has tangible/measurable components as well as aspects that are less tangible and relationship-based; and it is both dynamic and unstable.

Contextual antecedents

An antecedent is a preceding event or characteristic that leads to something else, in this case an effective context. It can be useful to know more about antecedents because it may be possible to intervene to alter the impact of a process on contextual attributes. The chapters in this book illustrate a broad and varied collection of antecedents that can impact on the characteristics of a practice context and these antecedents are consistent with those raised at the KU09 event.

Antecedents that are evident in this book and which are consistent with those raised at the KU09 event include:

- political/government priorities
- education and learning curricula and strategies
- interprofessional education and socialization
- adoption of a patient-centered perspective
- personal characteristics of individual clinicians
- resources, e.g., information technology and people
- staff development opportunities
- fit for purpose documentation
- effective leadership.

It is difficult to determine any clear relationship between these antecedents and whilst the authors contributing to this book place varying degrees of importance on different attributes, there is no clear evidence of determinants between the antecedents and the attributes. This is clearly an area requiring further research as it suggests that the factors that might most influence context are time and situation dependent. For example, the chapters of this book could be used as a data set to which a discourse analytical approach could be applied in order to tease out potential relationships and evaluate these through multiple case studies.

Common contextual factors

Building on the discussions arising from the KU09 meeting, and incorporating the contextual factors outlined in this book, it is clear that there are a number of common contextual factors that transcend settings. In Chapter 2 we explored the different levels at which contextual factors can impact or emerge as influencing factors on knowledge translation. These clearly begin to relate to and add some clarity to the concepts of Mode 2 knowledge articulated by Gibbons (2008). We make this assertion because whilst Gibbons' Mode 2 knowledge framework clearly demonstrates the importance of paying careful attention to the differing levels of context (micro-, meso-, and macro-levels), the meta-theoretical framework provided by Gibbons needs unpicking and careful deconstruction in order to develop its utility as a framework for decision making in knowledge utilization and translation activities. Trying to match contextual factors to their levels of significance at different organizational levels may be a fruitful activity and one that can help us tease out future priorities in knowledge utilization and translation studies. In Table 11.1 the common factors that emerged from KU09 and the chapters in this book have been mapped against the micro-, meso-, and macro-levels and again form the basis for further discussion.

Table 11.1 Common contextual factors by level of influence

| | Levels of action/effect | | | |
| | Micro | | Meso | Macro |
Contextual factors	Individual	Unit/team	Organizational	System
Readiness or willingness to change	✓	✓	✓	✓
Knowledge flow or exchange	✓	✓	✓	✓
Interpersonal interactions	✓	✓	✓	
Complexity of setting: e.g.,		✓	✓	
- Staff relationships				
- Acuity of patients				
- Skill-mix				
- Extent of family involvement in care				
- Multidisciplinary influences				
Attitudes/belief systems	✓	✓	✓	
Role clarity	✓	✓		
Physical environment		✓	✓	✓
Climate (level of background change)		✓	✓	✓
Culture		✓	✓	✓
Organizational slack		✓	✓	✓
Leadership		✓	✓	✓
Type of knowledge access (e.g., text, electronic)		✓	✓	✓

Considering these individual contexts—context within contexts

Taking the first two of these common factors, readiness to change and knowledge flow and exchange, the spread across the different levels have all been captured in the various chapters of this book. They also feature in several of the theories and models that have been developed to guide or explain the translation of evidence into practice (the first book in this series explores these in much more detail than we have been able to do). What is clear is that there are distinct spheres of influence at each level and each interacts with others. What we don't know is the strength or pattern of such interactions. One of the examples given in Chapter 5 reflects the issues related to readiness to change. The neonatal intensive care unit (or special care nursery as it may also be called) has a workforce made up of individuals, all of whom will see practice change in different ways and their personal readiness to change will vary from one person to another. Similarly the unit itself is a distinct entity, which reflects the culture of the larger organization but also of its members. This unit too must be ready to change, as must the larger organization. The PARIHS framework (Kitson et al., 2008; Rycroft-Malone, 2004) includes assessment of context and includes these factors.

The impact of the changing world on contextual factors for evidence-based healthcare?

The wider influences on healthcare delivery are many and varied and add further to the complexity of context. The changing world of healthcare presents practitioners with many challenges; one only needs to look at the issues that are now arising from the growth in information transfer through the Internet to get an idea of the size of the problem. Changes and growth should not always be seen negatively and so these challenges may not, in fact, be problems. However, they need to be understood in order for them to be managed effectively. The vast amount and array of knowledge that is communicated through technology today affects everyone from the user of healthcare to those who deliver it. Worldwide, there are still some countries where access to technology is poor, whilst others take it for granted. Strategies must be put in place to ensure that evidence is transferred in other formats. The Joanna Briggs Institute (JBI), based in Australia, established a program to support evidence-based practice centers linked to the Joanna Briggs Collaboration (for more information see http://www.joannabriggs.edu.au/about/ outreach-program.php) that do not have the same level of access to the electronic media that most of the other collaborating centers take for granted. The organization encourages and invites sponsorship that is used to establish and promote all-of-country access to www.jbiconnect.org for countries classified as having developing economies. In places where online access is poor, material is distributed via CD-ROM and this program is part of the organization's aim to support and facilitate evidence-based practice across the world.

Way forward

The dynamic nature of healthcare and the complexity of the contextual factors that are associated with healthcare today provide for an exciting but challenging future. There are developments taking place in the field of knowledge utilization and translation that will inevitably affect our understanding of context and the ways in which we implement and evaluate knowledge into practice. New models, such as that developed by Kontos and Poland (2009), are drawing on alternative sciences to guide our understanding of knowledge translation activities (Kontos and Poland's model explores critical realism and the arts, something that earlier models do not do). The exploration of contextual factors in this book has highlighted similarities and differences within and between settings. Some synthesis has begun to occur but more needs to be done to enable a greater understanding of context and its role in evidence implementation and practice change in the future. We do not know the strength of influence of the contextual factors identified in the PARIHS framework, or those that have been captured in this book. Therefore more research is needed to achieve this level of understanding.

The debate and discussions about context must continue to occur. We hope that we have presented ideas and examples and provided food for thought. The next wave of activity must occur in clinical settings such as those that we have included. We know that there are lots of others settings and specialist areas of practice that have other unique contextual influences—the discourse must also occur there.

It is no good to try to stop knowledge from going forward. Ignorance is never better than knowledge.

Enrico Fermi (1901–1954)

References

British Committee for Standards in Haematology, Blood Transfusion Task Force Royal College of Nursing & the Royal College of Surgeons of England (1999). The administration of blood and blood components and the management of transfused patients. *Transfusion Medicine*, 9, 227–239.

Gibbons, M. (2008). Why is knowedge translation important? Grounding the conversation. *Focus*. Available at http://www.ncddr.org/kt/products/focus/focus21/ (accessed May 25, 2009).

Gray-Micelli, D. (2008). Preventing falls in acute care. In: Capezuti, E., Zwicker, D., Mezey, M. & Fulmer, T. (eds) *Evidence-Based Geriatric Nursing Protocols for Best Practice*. New York (NY): Springer Publishing Company.

Kent, B., Hutchinson, A.M. & Fineout-Overholt, E. (2009). Getting evidence into practice—understanding knowledge translation to achieve practice change. *Worldviews on Evidence-Based Nursing*, 6, 183–185.

Kitson, A.L., Rycroft-Malone, J., Harvey, G., McCormack, B., Seers, K. & Titchen, A. (2008). Evaluating the successful implementation of evidence into practice using the PARIHS framework: Theoretical and practice challenges. *Implementation Science*, 3.

Kontos, P. & Poland, B. (2009). Mapping new theoretical and methodological terrain for knowledge translation: Contributions from critical realism and the arts. *Implementation Science*, 4.

McCormack, B. & Wright, J. (2009). Using the Context Assessment Index (CAI) in practice: Facilitating consciousness raising for practice development Newtownabbey, Co. Antrim: University of Ulster.

McCormack, B., Kitson, A., Harvey, G., Rycroft-Malone, J., Titchen, A. & Seers, K. (2002). Getting evidence into practice: The meaning of "context." *Journal of Advanced Nursing*, 38, 94–104.

Murphy, T., Labonte, P., Klock, M. & Houser, L. (2008). Falls prevention for elders in acute care—an evidence-based nursing practice initiative. *Critical Care Nursing Quarterly*, 31, 33–39.

Rycroft-Malone, J. (2004). The PARIHS framework—a framework for guiding the implementation of evidence-based practice. Promoting Action on Research Implementation in Health Services. *Journal of Nursing Care Quality*, 19, 297–304.

Taylor, C.J., Murphy, C.M.F., Lowe, D. & Pearson, M.M. (2008). Changes in practice and organisation surrounding blood transfusion in NHS trusts in England 1995–2005. *Quality and Safety in Health Care*, 17(4), 239–243.

Index